SAINT-FRANCES
⊢ GUIDE TO ⊢
CARDIOLOGY

SAINT-FRANCES GUIDE TO CARDIOLOGY

Andrew D. Michaels, M.D.

Assistant Professor of Clinical Medicine
Division of Interventional Cardiology
University of California, San Francisco
San Francisco, California

Craig Frances, M.D.

Clinical Instructor
University of California, San Francisco
San Francisco, California

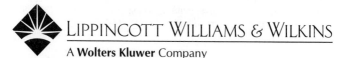

LIPPINCOTT WILLIAMS & WILKINS
A **Wolters Kluwer** Company

Philadelphia · Baltimore · New York · London
Buenos Aires · Hong Kong · Sydney · Tokyo

Editor: Elizabeth A. Nieginski
Editorial Director: Julie P. Scardiglia
Development Editor: Bridget Blatteau
Managing Editor: Marette Magargle-Smith
Marketing Manager: Kelley Ray

351 West Camden Street
Baltimore, Maryland 21201-2436 USA

530 Walnut Street
Philadelphia, Pennsylvania 19106 USA

Printed in the United States of America

Library of Congress Cataloging-in-Publication Data

Michaels, Andrew D.
   Saint-Frances guide to cardiology / Andrew D. Michaels, Craig Frances.
     p. cm.
   Includes index.
   ISBN 0-683-30660-X
   1. Cardiology—Outlines, syllabi, etc. 2. Heart—Diseases—Outlines, syllabi, etc. I. Frances, Craig. II. Title.

RC669 .M536 2000
616.1'2—dc21   00-056541

We'd like to hear from you! If you have comments or suggestions regarding this Lippincott Williams & Wilkins title, please contact us at the appropriate customer service number listed below, or send correspondence to **book_comments@lww.com.** If possible, please remember to include your mailing address, phone number, and a reference to the book title and author in your message. To purchase additional copies of this book call our customer service department at **(800) 638-3030** or fax orders to **(301) 824-7390.** International customers should call **(301) 714-2324.**

00 01 02
1 2 3 4 5 6 7 8 9 10

Dedication

To Renee, Rachel, and Matthew
and Mom, Dad, and Linda
Andrew D. Michaels

To Bob, Stacy, Tyler, and Olivia
Craig Frances

SAINT-FRANCES
GUIDE TO
CARDIOLOGY

Contents
✦

Preface

No field of medicine has experienced an explosion in knowledge in such a short period as cardiology has within the last decade. The field of cardiology is indeed overwhelming. As you progress in your education and your responsibilities increase, your anxiety level may also rise. As an intern and resident, you will often care for patients with complex and life-threatening disorders, but you may not have an approach to help you deal with the problems you encounter. Textbooks may not reduce your anxiety, because long lists of information are usually presented in a way that may not make sense or is too difficult to remember. Furthermore, patients usually do not present with easily defined diseases; rather, they present with symptoms and signs. By primarily addressing individual diseases, many texts work backward from what happens in real life.

Our book is meant to be very practical. We have found simple and straightforward approaches to common problems in cardiology that are easy to learn and equally easy to remember. To help you visually categorize the information, we provide you with algorithms, figures, and tables. We teach you how to approach patients in a step-by-step fashion. Some chapters, including those on syncope, chest pain, and dyspnea, provide you with ways to work forward from clinical presentation to diagnosis. Other chapters, like those on arrhythmias, heart failure, coronary disease, and valve disease, discuss the diagnoses you will make in greater depth. So, while you learn how to approach all patients with syncope, you will also learn the salient features of the causes of syncope (e.g., arrhythmias, valvular heart disease).

Additional chapters are provided to address other important topics in cardiology, such as congenital heart disease, drug interactions, pregnancy, geriatric cardiology, and perioperative cardiology. Appendices summarize key information, providing a quick reference for equations used in cardiology, cardiovascular drugs, and advanced cardiac life support (ACLS) protocols.

In many ways, the practice of cardiology is like a maze. The clinician is faced with a long row of doors, each of which may be opened, leading to another series of doors. *Saint-Frances Guide to Cardiology* is meant to help you consider the possible doors from the start so that you don't wander off in the wrong direction. We hope to guide you through the maze by helping you open the doors that lead to the correct diagnoses. While this book provides you with a concise review for the cardiology section of the internal medicine board examination, our ultimate goal is to help you take excellent care of your patients. In the process, we hope to make medicine manageable and fun.

Acknowledgments

We would like to acknowledge the cardiology faculty, fellows, house staff, and students at University of California, San Francisco, for making teaching so fulfilling. A special thanks goes to William Parmley, M.D., Tony Chou, M.D., Tom Ports, M.D., William Grossman, M.D., Lee Goldman, M.D., Joel Karliner, M.D., Gregory Schwartz, M.D., PhD, and Tom Evans, M.D. for their mentorship and guidance. We would like to acknowledge Elizabeth Nieginski for her critical role in helping to create the Saint-Frances guides. We would also like to thank our editor, Bridget Blatteau, whose tireless and talented input is greatly appreciated. Finally, we wish to thank our families for their unwavering support.

PART 1

ASSESSMENT AND DIAGNOSTIC TESTING

1. Cardiac Examination

I **NECK VEIN EXAMINATION.** Examination of the neck veins is an underutilized yet important part of the cardiac examination. With practice, an accurate determination of the central venous pressure (CVP) and waveforms can be obtained.

A. **Patient positioning**. The patient should sit upright at an approximately 30° elevation, with the clinician standing on the patient's right side. The bed angle may need to be raised or lowered until the crests of the venous pulsations can be seen. The patient's head should be kept midline; the common mistake of turning the head to the left results in contraction of the right sternocleidomastoid muscle and an obscured view. A penlight often can highlight the veins tangentially (i.e., from front to back).

B. **Anatomy**
   1. **Internal jugular veins. The right internal jugular vein** best displays the various waveforms because of its direct route to the right atrium. The internal jugular vein travels in a straight line from the jugular notch in the medial edge of the clavicle to the mastoid process behind the ear.
   2. **External jugular veins** may be used if the internal jugular veins cannot be appreciated. Because the external jugular veins have one-way valves, a difference in the "pulsating meniscus" level between the internal and external jugular veins can distinguish elevated venous pressure from the retrograde flow of tricuspid regurgitation. If the CVP in the internal jugular vein is higher than the CVP in the external jugular vein, suspect tricuspid regurgitation.
   3. **Carotid arteries.** The carotid impulse can be timed with the first heart sound (S_1), which occurs slightly before the pulsation. Placing the side of the hand against the base of the neck obstructs jugular pulsations, but the carotid impulses are usually unchanged.

C. Findings
1. CVP
a. To estimate the CVP, hold a straight edge from the crest of the jugular venous pulsation horizontally across to the point above the sternal angle. Measure the vertical distance from the straight edge to the sternal angle, and add 5 centimeters.

(1) A **CVP < 8 cm H$_2$O** is considered normal.

(2) A **CVP ≥ 8 cm H$_2$O** may be found with right or left ventricular failure, tricuspid stenosis, cardiac tamponade, and constrictive pericarditis.

b. When the CVP is greatly elevated, the patient's earlobe may pulsate or the veins on the top of the head may become distended.

2. Waveforms
a. Venous. Simultaneous palpation of the left carotid artery and visualization of the venous pulsations help the examiner relate the venous pulsations to the timing of the cardiac cycle (Figure 1-1).

(1) The presystolic *a* **wave** is produced by right atrial contraction.

(2) The *c* **wave** is produced during right ventricular sys-

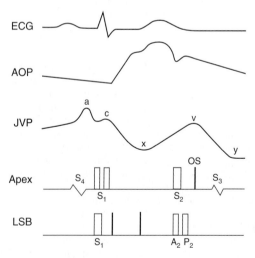

FIGURE 1-1. Simultaneous recordings of the electrocardiogram (*ECG*), aortic pressure (*AOP*), jugular venous pulsations (*JVP*), and heart tones heard at the apex and left sternal border (*LSB*). *OS* indicates the opening snap.

tole with bulging of the tricuspid valve into the right atrium.

   (3) The x **descent** follows the c wave and is caused by atrial relaxation.

   (4) The late systolic v **wave** peaks when the tricuspid valve opens.

   (5) The y descent follows and is related to atrial emptying of blood into the right ventricle.

  b. Arterial. The arterial pulse wave has a smooth, rapid upstroke and a dome-shaped summit (see Figure 1-1).

   (1) The **bisferious pulse** ("twice-beating") is seen in hypertrophic cardiomyopathy and also in aortic regurgitation alone or combined with aortic stenosis.

   (2) The **dicrotic pulse** refers to a palpable diastolic pulse seen in low-output cardiac states.

II PRECORDIAL PALPATION

A. Technique. The **point of maximal impulse (PMI)** is normally appreciated in the fourth or fifth interspaces of the left midclavicular line.

B. Findings

  1. Normally, the examiner feels the impulse hit and leave the fingers before feeling the carotid impulse with the other hand.

  2. A **sustained left ventricular impulse (i.e., heave)** is diagnosed when there is overlap with the carotid impulse, and it indicates **left ventricular hypertrophy** or **dilatation** (i.e., failure). The following assessments can be used to distinguish between hypertrophy and dilatation.

   a. Location. Displacement of the PMI inferolaterally indicates dilatation.

   b. Size. A PMI greater than the size of a quarter indicates dilatation.

   c. Kinetics. Dilatation usually causes a hypokinetic PMI, whereas hypertrophy results in a hyperkinetic PMI.

   d. Gallops. A palpable third heart sound (S_3) is usually associated with dilatation, whereas a fourth heart sound (S_4) usually indicates hypertrophy.

III AUSCULTATION

A. Technique

  1. The **areas where each valve is best heard** are listed in Figure 1-2.

   a. The diaphragm of the stethoscope is used to evaluate normal heart sounds, murmurs, and clicks.

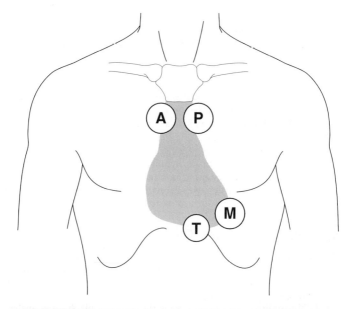

Valve	Portion of Stethoscope	Positioning
Aortic (A)	Diaphragm	Right sternal border, 2nd interspace
Pulmonic (P)	Diaphragm	Left sternal border, 2nd interspace
Tricuspid (T)	Bell	Left lower sternal border
Mitral (M)	Bell	Apex and left lower sternal border

FIGURE 1-2. Auscultation of the heart valves.

    b. The bell is used to detect low-pitched sounds (i.e., gallops).
  2. A frequently used **pattern of auscultation** is to start with the diaphragm of the stethoscope at the base of the heart (i.e., the aortic and pulmonic areas), focusing on the S_1 and second heart sound (S_2), and then any accompanying murmurs. Then move down the left lower sternal border and over to the apex. At the apex, use the bell of the stethoscope to listen for gallops.
B. Findings. Rather than trying to appreciate all normal and abnormal sounds simultaneously, direct your attention to the S_1, then to the S_2, and finally to murmurs.

1. **"Split" S_1.** If you hear two components of the S_1, the main differential diagnoses include an S_4 and a split S_1.
   a. The following assessments can help you distinguish between a split S_1 and an S_4.
      (1) **Location.** The tricuspid valve is usually quiet because it is closed by a low-pressure system. Hearing two sounds over the tricuspid area favors a split S_1, while hearing two sounds over the apex favors an S_4.
      (2) **Pitch.** An S_4 is low-pitched and best heard with the bell of the stethoscope, whereas the tricuspid sound (T_1) is high-pitched and best heard with the diaphragm.
      (3) **Volume.** Closure of the mitral valve is usually louder than an S_4 or T_1. If the first of the two "split" sounds is louder, mitral valve closure followed by T_1 is more likely. A louder second sound favors an S_4 followed by closure of the mitral valve.
   b. After distinguishing between a split S_1 and an S_4, the clinician may be able to narrow the diagnosis.
      (1) A **widely split S_1** is seen in right bundle branch block (RBBB), ectopic beats, mitral stenosis, left atrial myxoma, and Ebstein's anomaly.
      (2) An **S_4** is caused by a high velocity atrial kick, and is seen in the setting of a noncompliant ventricle [e.g., in left ventricular hypertrophy (LVH), aortic stenosis, or myocardial ischemia].
2. **"Split" S_2.** If you hear two components of the S_2, the differential diagnoses include an **S_3**, a **split S_2**, and, rarely, a **pericardial knock** in constrictive pericarditis.
   a. The following assessments can help you distinguish between an S_3 and a split S_2.
      (1) **Location.** An S_3 is usually best heard over the apex or the left lower sternal border, depending on whether the sound is emanating from the left or right ventricle. A split S_2 is best heard in the left third intercostal space (i.e., Erb's point).
      (2) **Pitch.** An S_3 is very low pitched and heard only with the bell, whereas pulmonic closure causes a higher pitched sound that is best heard with the diaphragm.
      (3) **Changes with respiration.** While an S_3 is unlikely to change with the respiratory cycle, a split S_2 may have respiratory variations that cause the intermittent appearance and disappearance of one of the S_2 sounds.
   b. After distinguishing between a split S_2 and an S_3, the clinician may be able to narrow the diagnosis.
      (1) **Expiratory splitting of the S_2** is often caused by pulmonic stenosis, RBBB, atrial septal defect (ASD),

ventricular septal defect (VSD), and pulmonary hypertension.

(2) A **single S₂** may be heard in aortic stenosis, left bundle branch block (LBBB), tricuspid atresia, and tetralogy of Fallot.

(3) An **S₃** is often seen in severe mitral regurgitation and congestive heart failure (CHF), conditions in which increased early mitral flow is present.

3. **Murmurs** are either innocent, systolic (between S_1 and S_2), diastolic (after S_2), or continuous (beginning in systole and continuing into diastole without interruption). Simultaneously palpating the carotid artery during auscultation can help you categorize the timing of the murmurs.

   a. **Innocent murmurs** are usually short, often modified by respiration, and associated with a normal S_2. In most cases, they are not loud, nor are they holosystolic or diastolic. Innocent murmurs are often produced by **high output states** (e.g., sepsis, anemia, pregnancy, thyrotoxicosis).

   b. **Systolic murmurs** can be classified as holosystolic, midsystolic, or late systolic. The maneuvers for assessing a systolic murmur, along with their associated findings, are listed in Table 1-1.

      (1) **Holosystolic murmurs** begin at S_1 and end at S_2. Holosystolic murmurs are often associated with the following disorders.

         (a) **Mitral regurgitation** produces a murmur that is loudest at the apex, usually radiates to the axilla, and does not increase with inspiration. If a flail posterior leaflet causes the murmur, the sound may radiate to the base.

         (b) **Tricuspid regurgitation** produces a murmur that is best heard over the tricuspid area, increases with inspiration, and may be associated with prominent *v* waves.

         (c) **VSD** produces a murmur that is best heard at the left lower sternal border, often radiates to the right sternal border, and does not increase with inspiration. The intensity of the murmur will increase when the patient squeezes a fist (i.e., the hand grip maneuver).

      (2) **Midsystolic murmurs** begin after S_1 and end prior to S_2.

         (a) **Aortic stenosis** produces a harsh, crescendo-decrescendo midsystolic murmur that is usually best heard at the aortic area, often radiates to the carotid arteries, and does not change with respi-

TABLE 1-1. Systolic Murmur Maneuvers

Maneuver	Venous Return	Arterial Resistance	Murmur Intensity	Possible Cause of Murmur
Standing to squatting	Increased	Increased	Decreased	HOCM
				Mitral valve prolapse
Lifting of legs	Increased	Increased	Decreased	HOCM
				Mitral valve prolapse
	Increased	Increased	Increased	Aortic stenosis
Hand grip	Unchanged	Increased	Increased	Mitral regurgitation
				VSD
Inspiration	Increased	Unchanged	Increased	Tricuspid regurgitation
				Pulmonic stenosis
Valsalva	Decreased	Increased	Decreased	Aortic stenosis
	Decreased	Increased	Increased	HOCM

HOCM = hypertrophic obstructive cardiomyopathy, VSD = ventricular septal defect.

7

ration. As the stenosis becomes more severe, the peaking of the murmur occurs later in systole, and the aortic component of the second heart sound (A_2) becomes softer.

- **(b) Aortic sclerosis** is common in the elderly and is often difficult to differentiate from aortic stenosis. A normal S_1, loud A_2, and early peaking of the murmur, along with a normal carotid upstroke, usually indicate aortic sclerosis.
- **(c) Hypertrophic obstructive cardiomyopathy (HOCM)** may result in left ventricular outflow obstruction, producing a murmur that can be distinguished from aortic stenosis because it decreases with passive leg lifting and on changing position from standing to squatting. The intensity of the murmurs from HOCM increases during inspiration.
- **(d) Pulmonic stenosis,** which is rare in adults, produces a murmur that is best heard over the pulmonic area and increases with inspiration.
- **(3) Late systolic murmurs** begin after S_1 and end at S_2, and usually imply **mitral valve prolapse**. A click may precede the murmur. Decreasing the left ventricular volume (e.g., by performing a Valsalva maneuver) will cause the click to occur earlier and lengthen the murmur.
- **c. Diastolic murmurs** can be similarly classified, as early diastolic, mid-diastolic, or late diastolic.
  - **(1) Early diastolic murmurs**
    - **(a) Aortic insufficiency** results in a decrescendo murmur over the aortic area. It is best heard with the patient sitting upright, leaning forward, and holding her breath at end-expiration. A very short, soft murmur may indicate acute aortic insufficiency because the left ventricle is nondistensible and prevents blood from rushing back into the ventricle from the aorta.
    - **(b) Pulmonic insufficiency** produces a **Graham Steell's murmur** that is best heard over the pulmonic area. This murmur is similar in quality and location to that of aortic insufficiency. This murmur is most commonly seen secondary to pulmonary hypertension, and can be distinguished from aortic insufficiency by its louder intensity with inspiration.
  - **(2) Mid-diastolic murmurs**
    - **(a) Mitral stenosis** often causes an early diastolic,

high-frequency opening snap followed by a subtle rumble. Listen for the murmur at the apex, with the patient in the left lateral decubitus position.

   (b) Tricuspid stenosis is best heard over the tricuspid area and increases with inspiration.

   (3) Late diastolic murmurs usually represent **mitral** or **tricuspid stenosis**.

   d. Continuous murmurs are less common in adults. Pathologic conditions that cause these murmurs include the following.

   (1) Patent ductus arteriosus (PDA) results in the classic **"machinery" murmur.**

   (2) Coarctation of the aorta may produce a continuous murmur that is best heard over the back.

   (3) Arteriovenous fistulae (systemic, pulmonary, and coronary), whether iatrogenic or congenital, may also result in continuous murmurs.

References

Chatterjee K: Bedside evaluation of the heart: the physical examination. In *Cardiology: Physiology, Pharmacology, Diagnosis.* Edited by Parmley WW, Chatterjee K. New York, Lippincott-Raven, 1995, pp 1–55.

O'Rourke RA, Shaver JA, Salerni R, et al: The history, physical examination, and cardiac auscultation. In *Hurst's The Heart,* 9th ed. Edited by Alexander RW, Schlant RC, Foster V. New York, McGraw-Hill, 1998, pp 229–342.

2. Electrocardiogram Interpretation

....

I **INTRODUCTION.** There is no absolute right order for in-
terpreting electrocardiograms (ECGs), but it is important to
choose a method and interpret each ECG precisely the same
way. One common approach is to evaluate ECG findings in
the following order: rhythm, rate, axis, intervals, hypertrophy, Q waves, and ST/T wave changes.

II RHYTHM

A. **Normal sinus rhythm.** If each normal P wave (atrial depolarization) is followed by a QRS complex (ventricular depolarization), and the heart rate is between 60 and 100 beats/min, then
the patient is in normal sinus rhythm. Sinus P waves are usually
upright in leads I, II, and aVF.
B. **Atrial rhythms** are characterized by nonsinus P waves (usually
not upright in leads I, II, and aVF) preceding each QRS complex and a heart rate between 60 and 100 beats/min.
   1. **Ectopic atrial rhythms** have nonsinus P waves preceding
   each QRS complex.
   2. **Multiform atrial rhythms** have at least 2 different, nonsinus
   P waveforms preceding each QRS complex and a heart rate
   between 60 and 100 beats/min.
C. **Bradycardia** is a heart rate less than 60 beats/min.
   1. **Sinus bradycardia.** Each QRS complex is preceded by a sinus P wave.
   2. Other forms of bradycardia [e.g., atrioventricular (AV)
   nodal block] are discussed in Section V A 2.
D. **Tachycardia** is a heart rate greater than 100 beats/min (see
Chapters 7 and 9).

III RATE

A. **Regular rhythm.** If the patient is in sinus rhythm, the easiest way
to calculate the heart rate is to divide 300 by the number of large
boxes between two successive QRS complexes (Table 2-1).
(Each large box is composed of five small boxes, each representing 0.04 second.)
B. **Irregular rhythm.** If the patient has an irregular rhythm, divide
several (e.g., 4–6) consecutive QRS complexes by the number

TABLE 2-1. Using the ECG to Determine Heart Rate for Patients in Sinus Rhythm*

Number of Large Boxes	Corresponding Heart Rate (beats/min)
1	300
2	150
3	100
4	75

Reprinted with permission from Saint S, Frances C: *Saint-Frances Guide to Inpatient Medicine.* Media, PA, Williams & Wilkins, 1997, p 22.

*Divide 300 by the number of large boxes between two successive QRS complexes.

of large boxes between them to get the average time between the QRS complexes. Divide 300 by this average to get the heart rate.

C. Bradycardia. If the patient's heart rate is very slow, multiply the number of QRS complexes seen on one sheet of the ECG (each page on the usual paper speed of 25 mm/sec records 10 seconds) by six. (Ten-second periods are equivalent to 50 large boxes.)

IV **AXIS.** The QRS axis is the net vector generated by all ventricular depolarization. While the exact axis is not clinically useful, it is important to determine whether the axis is normal, shifted left, or shifted right. Left and right axis shifts usually suggest disease of the ventricular myocardium.

A. Axis characteristics
   1. A **normal axis** is between −30° and +90°.
   2. A **leftward axis** is more negative than −30°. It also can be called a superior axis (because it is moving left toward the 12 o'clock position).
   3. A **rightward axis** is more positive than +90°.
B. Determining axis (Figure 2-1)
   1. **Normal axis.** Both leads I and II are positive.
   2. **Leftward axis.** Lead I is positive and lead II is negative.
   3. **Rightward axis.** Lead I is negative and lead II is positive.
   4. **Right superior axis.** Both leads I and II are negative.
C. Causes of axis deviation
   1. **Left axis deviation (LAD).** Left anterior fascicular block and inferior wall myocardial infarction (MI) account for most cases of LAD.
      a. Left anterior fascicular block (LAFB)
         (1) Pathogenesis. The left bundle splits into anterior and

A

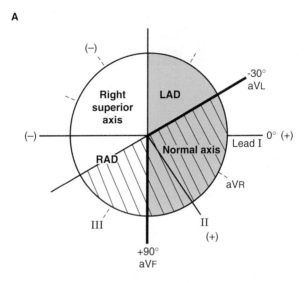

B

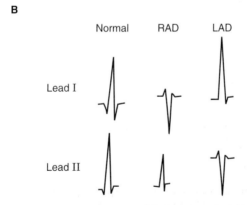

FIGURE 2-1. *(A)* Determining axis. If the QRS complex of lead I is net positive (i.e., the area above the horizontal is greater than the area below), the axis must lie somewhere in the *gray shaded* region. If lead II is net positive, then the axis must lie in the *cross-hatched* region. The area of overlap denotes the range for a normal axis. *(B)* Appearance of the QRS complex in leads I and II in left axis deviation (LAD), right axis deviation (RAD), and normal axis. (Reprinted with permission from Saint S, Frances C: *Saint-Frances Guide to Inpatient Medicine.* Media, PA, Williams & Wilkins, 1997, p 23.)

posterior fascicles, with the anterior fascicle running superiorly. When the anterior fascicle is blocked, the muscle that it serves must be depolarized from inferior forces. These "extra" inferior to superior-directed forces rotate the axis leftward.

(2) **Criteria for diagnosis** include an axis between $-45°$ and $-90°$, a QR pattern in lead aVL, an R peak time (from the beginning of the Q to the peak of the R) in lead aVL greater than or equal to 45 msec, and a QRS complex less than 0.12 second in duration.

(3) **Conditions causing LAFB** include hypertensive heart disease, coronary artery disease (CAD), and idiopathic conducting system disease.

b. **Inferior wall MI**

(1) **Pathogenesis.** Infarcted myocardium at the inferior aspect of the left ventricle does not conduct; therefore, more net forces are directed superiorly (or leftward).

(2) **Criteria for diagnosis** include pathologic Q waves ($>$ 30 msec in duration) in leads II and aVF.

c. **Posteroseptal accessory pathway (Wolff-Parkinson-White syndrome).** Look for negative delta waves in the inferior leads, a short PR interval ($<$ 0.12 second in duration), and a tall R wave in lead V_2.

d. **Chronic obstructive pulmonary disease (COPD).** A lower diaphragm can move the right ventricle below the larger left ventricle, resulting in more forces directed superiorly. When accompanied by pulmonary hypertension, however, COPD often produces right axis deviation (RAD).

e. **Congenital heart disease** (e.g., atrial or ventricular septal defect) can also cause LAD.

2. **Right axis deviation (RAD)**

a. **Right ventricular hypertrophy (RVH).** RAD is caused by RVH until proven otherwise. (Criteria for RVH are discussed in Section VI B.)

b. **Acute cor pulmonale** (e.g., pulmonary embolus, acute bronchospasm). Look for a rightward shift of the axis of more than 30° when compared with a prior ECG.

c. **Lateral MI.** Look for pathologic Q waves ($\geq$ 30 msec in duration) in leads I and aVL.

d. **Left ventricular free-wall accessory pathway (Wolff-Parkinson-White syndrome).** Look for a short PR interval and a positive delta wave in lead V_1.

e. **Left posterior fascicular block (LPFB).** Consider this a diagnosis of exclusion.

f. **Limb lead reversal.** Look for an inverted P wave in lead I.

g. **Pneumothorax**

h. **Tricyclic antidepressant overdose.** Look for first-degree

AV nodal block, widened QRS complexes, and prolonged
QT intervals.

V INTERVALS

A. PR interval. The PR interval is normally between 0.12 and 0.20
second in duration. The appropriate measurement is from the
beginning of the P wave to the beginning of the Q wave.
  1. A **short PR interval** is often caused by a high catecholamine
     state that makes the AV node conduct faster; however, you
     should look for delta waves to exclude an accessory pathway.
  2. A **prolonged PR interval** is associated with increased vagal
     tone or permanent disease to the **conduction system.**
     a. **First-degree AV nodal block** is diagnosed if each P wave
        is followed by a QRS complex at a longer than normal in-
        terval (PR interval > 0.20 second in duration).
     b. **Second-degree AV nodal block** is diagnosed if some P
        waves are not followed by a QRS complex.
        (1) Mobitz type I block (Wenckebach block) is charac-
            terized by progressive prolongation of the PR inter-
            vals until a QRS complex is dropped.
        (2) Mobitz type II block is characterized by no variation
            in the PR intervals, with occasional dropping of the
            QRS complexes. There is a relatively fixed ratio of P
            waves to QRS complexes (e.g., 2:1, 3:2, or 4:3).
     c. **Third-degree AV nodal block.** P waves and QRS com-
        plexes are completely unrelated. The P-P interval is
        shorter than the R-R interval. The R-R interval is regular.
B. QRS interval. The QRS interval is normally less than 0.10 second in duration. Measurement is from the beginning of the Q
wave to the end of the S wave.
  1. **Interventricular conduction delay** or **incomplete bundle
     branch block** is diagnosed when the QRS interval is
     0.10–0.12 second in duration.
  2. **Bundle branch block** is diagnosed when the QRS interval is
     greater than 0.12 second in duration ("widened").
     a. **Pathogenesis**
        (1) Right bundle branch block (RBBB). If the right bun-
            dle is blocked, depolarization must proceed down the
            left bundle and then slowly to the right from muscle
            fiber to muscle fiber. Muscle conducts more slowly
            than the specialized conduction bundles; therefore,
            the QRS complex will be wider than normal, and the
            late electrical forces will move to the right.
        (2) Left bundle branch block (LBBB). If the left bundle is
            blocked, a similar reaction occurs, the QRS complex
            will widen, and the late forces will move to the left.

b. Diagnosis

    (1) Determine the direction of the late forces (Figure 2-2). Draw a line down the middle of the QRS complex in leads V_1 (a rightward lead) and V_6 (a leftward lead). The half of the QRS complex to the right of the line represents the "late" forces. Check if these are positive (above the horizontal) or negative (below the horizontal).

    (2) Interpret the late forces

        (a) RBBB. If the late forces of V_1 are positive and those of V_6 are negative, then the late forces are moving from the left toward the right, signifying an RBBB.

        (b) LBBB. If the late forces of V_6 are positive and those of V_1 are negative, then the late forces are moving from the right toward the left, signifying an LBBB.

        (c) Nonspecific interventricular bundle branch block is often diagnosed when the late forces of V_1 and V_6 are either both positive or both negative.

A. Right bundle branch block

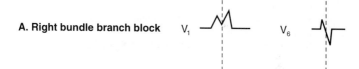

B. Left bundle branch block

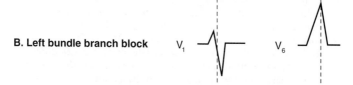

FIGURE 2-2. Determining the direction of the late forces. *(A)* Right bundle branch block. The late forces are positive in lead V_1 and negative in lead V_6. *(B)* Left bundle branch block. The late forces are negative in lead V_1 and positive in lead V_6. (Reprinted with permission from Saint S, Frances C: *Saint-Frances Guide to Inpatient Medicine.* Media, PA, Williams & Wilkins, 1997, p 27.)

C. QT interval. The QT interval varies according to the **heart rate.** The QT interval is normally between 0.3 and 0.48 second in duration. Measurement is from the beginning of the Q wave to the end of the T wave. The QT interval is best recorded in leads V_2 and V_3.

1. **Prolonged QT interval.** A QT interval greater than 0.48 second in duration is almost always abnormal. Drugs (e.g., tricyclic antidepressants, amiodarone, type Ia antiarrhythmics) and electrolyte abnormalities (e.g., hypokalemia, hypomagnesemia, hypocalcemia) are common causes of prolonged QT interval.

2. **Short QT interval.** A QT interval shorter than 0.3 second in duration is usually abnormal, but it can be seen in patients with tachycardia. Causes of a short QT interval include drugs (e.g., digoxin) and electrolyte abnormalities (e.g., hypercalcemia).

VI HYPERTROPHY

A. Left ventricular hypertrophy (LVH). All ECG criteria for the diagnosis of LVH are highly specific but poorly sensitive. One approach is to proceed through the following criteria in the order given. If a criterion is met, you diagnose LVH; if not, you move to the next criterion.

1. **R wave in lead aVL** greater than 11 mm (> 13 mm if LAFB is present)
2. **R wave in lead aVL + S wave in lead V_3** greater than 20 mm in a woman or 28 mm in a man
3. **S wave in lead V_1 + R wave in lead V_5 or V_6** (whichever is larger) greater than 35 mm

B. RVH. Criteria for the diagnosis of RVH are also highly specific but poorly sensitive.

1. **R:S wave ratio in lead V_1** greater than or equal to 1
2. **R wave in lead V_1** greater than 7 mm
3. **R:S wave ratio in lead V_5 or V_6** less than 1
4. **S wave in V_5 or V_6** greater than 7 mm

C. Left atrial abnormality (LAA) formerly was called left atrial enlargement, but the name was changed because the ECG findings may actually represent an increase in left atrial size, pressure, or wall thickness.

1. **Lead V_1.** If the terminal P force (the negative deflection that represents left atrial depolarization) is greater than or equal to 1 small box by 1 small box (0.04 sec by 1 mm), LAA is diagnosed.
2. **Lead II.** Notched P waves greater than 0.04 second apart (1 small box) indicate LAA.

D. Right atrial abnormality (RAA)

1. **Lead V_1 or V_2.** A P wave greater than 1.5 mm high indicates RAA.
2. **Lead II.** A P wave greater than 2.5 mm high indicates RAA.

VII **Q WAVES** simply indicate that forces are moving away from their respective leads.

A. Normal Q waves. Sometimes Q waves are normal and expected. For example, the interventricular septum is depolarized left to right, and so a Q wave is expected in lead V_6 (reflecting forces moving away from this leftward lead).

B. Pathologic Q waves signify that forces are moving away from the area more than would normally be expected. A pathologic Q wave indicates an **MI,** and is diagnosed when the Q wave is at least 30 msec (close to one small box) in duration and one-third the height of the ensuing R wave.

    1. An **anterior wall MI** is characterized by any Q waves in leads V_2 through V_4. A Q wave in V_1 alone can be normal.

        a. Lateral extension. An **anterolateral infarction** is an anterior wall MI that has additional Q waves in lead I or aVL.

        b. Apical extension. An **anteroapical infarction** is an anterior wall MI that has additional Q waves in leads V_5 and V_6.

    2. An **inferior wall MI** is characterized by pathologic Q waves in lead II or aVF. An isolated Q wave in lead III may be normal.

        a. Posterior extension. A **posterior wall MI** sometimes accompanies an inferior wall MI, producing a large R wave in lead V_1 or V_2. The differential diagnoses for a large R wave in V_1 or V_2 include:

        (1) Posterior wall MI
        (2) RVH
        (3) Posteroseptal accessory pathway
        (4) Right interventricular conduction delay
        (5) RBBB
        (6) Limb lead reversal
        (7) Dextrocardia
        (8) Duchenne's muscular dystrophy
        (9) Normal variant

        b. Lateral extension. An inferolateral infarction is an inferior wall MI that has additional Q waves in lead I or aVL.

VIII **ST/T WAVE CHANGES**

A. Terminology. Clinicians often refer to ST depressions and elevations as ischemia and infarct, respectively, rather than simply "injury." This is because **ST depression** is caused by injury to the **subendocardial** (inner) region of the myocardial wall, resulting from a supply and demand mismatch (e.g., ischemia). **ST elevation** implies **transmural** (full thickness) injury that usually occurs as a result of complete coronary occlusion during an acute myocardial infarction (AMI).

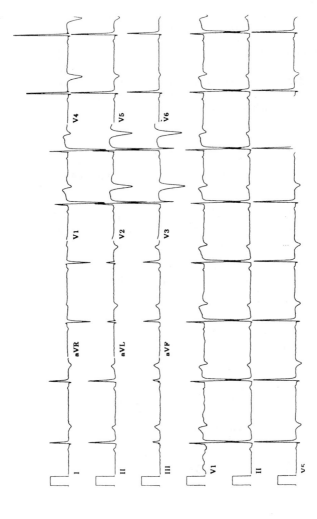

FIGURE 2-3. 12-lead electrocardiogram (ECG) of a 70-year-old man admitted with unstable angina. The large symmetric T wave inversions in leads V₂ through V₅ are caused by anterior wall myocardial ischemia. (Courtesy of G. Thomas Evans Jr., M.D., University of California San Francisco, San Francisco, CA)

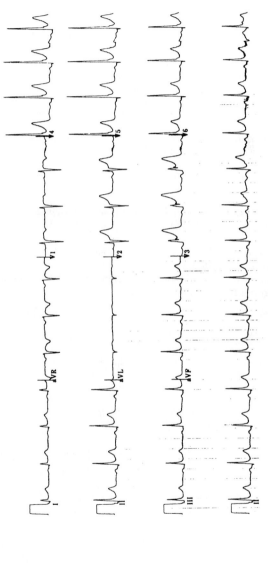

FIGURE 2-4. 12-lead electrocardiogram (ECG) of a 57-year-old man admitted with atypical chest pain. The ECG shows the characteristic appearance of ST elevation (narrow QRS complexes, tall R waves in the chest leads, and a distinct notch or slur in the downstroke of the R waves) in leads V_3 through V_6 often caused by early repolarization normal variant. (Courtesy of G. Thomas Evans Jr., M.D., University of California San Francisco, San Francisco, CA)

B. Causes. The most common causes of ST/T wave changes are:
1. **Myocardial ischemia** (Figure 2-3), **injury,** or **infarction**
2. **Ventricular enlargement**
3. **Abnormal ventricular depolarization** (e.g., with bundle branch block)
4. **Electrolyte disturbances** (hypo- or hyperkalemia, hypo- or hypercalcemia)
5. **Drugs** (class Ia antiarrhythmics, digoxin)
6. **Pericarditis** (See Chapter 21, Figure 21-1)
7. **Early repolarization normal variant** (Figure 2-4)

HOT

An old MI with a ventricular aneurysm can have persistent ST elevations, mimicking an AMI.

KEY

C. Findings
1. **T wave inversions** often indicate **myocardial ischemia.** Giant symmetric T wave inversions also can be seen in subarachnoid hemorrhage.
2. **ST depressions** often represent **subendocardial** ischemia.
3. **ST elevations** often represent **transmural** myocardial infarct. Diffuse ST elevations with depressions of the PR interval are often caused by acute pericarditis.

References

Castellanos A, Kessler KM, Myerburg RJ: The resting electrocardiogram. In *Hurst's The Heart,* 9th ed. Edited by Alexander RW, Schlant RC, Fuster V. New York: McGraw-Hill, 1998, pp 351–386.

Chou TC: *Electrocardiography in Clinical Practice: Adult and Pediatric,* 4th ed. Philadelphia, WB Saunders, 1996.

3. Approach to Diagnostic Testing

I **INTRODUCTION.** The probability of a disease is a continuum:

Probability of Disease

0% ———————————————————— 100%

Disease absent   Disease present

A. Many diseases listed on an initial differential diagnosis fall somewhere in the middle of this continuum.
B. The goal of the physician is to use the patient's history, examination, and diagnostic tests to move most diagnoses as far to the left as possible (reasonably excluding them), while moving one diagnosis as far to the right as possible.
C. The inappropriate use of diagnostic tests will leave many diagnoses frustratingly close to the midpoint of the continuum.

II **GOALS OF TESTING**

A. **Screening.** Diagnostic tests can help screen asymptomatic people for clinically silent disease. Screening is most beneficial when the following criteria are met:
   1. The **population** has a high prevalence of disease.
   2. The **disease** has significant morbidity and mortality and a presymptomatic period. In addition, effective treatment is available and, if initiated in the early stages, can help improve outcome.
   3. The **test** has good sensitivity and specificity and is inexpensive, well tolerated, and safe.
B. **Diagnosis.** In symptomatic patients, diagnostic tests can help establish or exclude the presence of a disease.
C. **Patient management.** Diagnostic tests can also be used to:
   1. Evaluate the severity of the disease and estimate prognosis.
   2. Monitor the course of the disease (e.g., progression, resolution, recurrence).
   3. Select and adjust therapy.

III TEST CHARACTERISTICS

A. Accuracy is a characteristic that compares a test's result to the true value (Figure 3-1).

B. Precision is a characteristic that measures the reproducibility of a test's results when the test is repeated under identical conditions (see Figure 3-1).

C. Sensitivity is the likelihood that a patient with disease has a positive test. A test with a high sensitivity (close to 100%) is useful to exclude a diagnosis because a highly sensitive test will have very few false-negative results.

D. Specificity is the likelihood that a healthy patient has a negative test. A test with a high specificity (close to 100%) is useful to confirm a diagnosis because a highly specific test will have very few false-positive results.

IV USING DIAGNOSTIC TESTS

A. The **pretest probability** is the probability of disease prior to testing.

   1. Consider the following three examples:

   a. A 45-year-old man presents to an urgent care clinic with a 2-month history of paroxysmal, sharp, left-sided chest pain occurring both at rest and with exercise. A literature search reveals that one-half of 45-year-old men with **atypical chest pain** have coronary artery disease (CAD). Therefore, the pretest probability of CAD in this patient is 50%.

   b. If the patient is a 30-year-old woman with atypical chest pain, the pretest probability of CAD would be 5%.

   c. If the patient is a 60-year-old man with exertional chest tightness **(typical angina),** the pretest probability of CAD would be 95%.

   2. Suppose all three of these patients undergo an exercise treadmill test. In order to determine whether a positive test

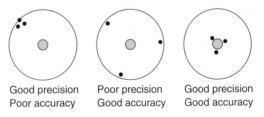

| Good precision | Poor precision | Good precision |
| Poor accuracy | Good accuracy | Good accuracy |

FIGURE 3-1. Relationship between accuracy and precision in testing. The center of the circle represents the truth.

rules in CAD and whether a negative test rules out CAD, it is necessary to consider the likelihood ratio (LR).

B. The **LR** is the strength of the diagnostic test result.
   1. The LR helps answer these clinically important questions:
      a. Given a positive test result, how likely is it that the disease is truly present?
      b. Given a negative test result, how likely is it that the disease is truly absent?
   2. Mathematically, a positive LR (LR^+) is the odds of having the disease given a positive test result versus not having the disease given a positive test result.

$LR^+ =$

$$\frac{\text{The chance of a positive test and disease}}{\text{The chance of a positive test and no disease}} = \frac{\text{(Sensitivity)}}{\text{(1 - Specificity)}}$$

A negative LR (LR^-) is the odds of having the disease given a negative test result versus not having the disease given a negative test result.

$LR^- =$

$$\frac{\text{The chance of a negative test and disease}}{\text{The chance of a negative test and no disease}} = \frac{\text{(1 - Sensitivity)}}{\text{(Specificity)}}$$

   a. For example, if 100 patients have a positive test and 75 actually have disease, then the LR^+ is 3. This number can be calculated using the following formula:

$$\frac{\text{The chance of a positive test and disease}}{\text{The chance of a positive test and no disease}} = \frac{75}{25} = \frac{3}{1}$$

   b. Consider another example. The LR^+ of a positive treadmill test is 3.5. In a large, heterogeneous population of patients, all of whom have had positive treadmill tests, 7 patients will actually have CAD for every 2 patients who do not. Therefore, if your patient has a positive treadmill test, the odds of that person having CAD are 7 to 2, or 3.5 to 1. That is, given a positive treadmill test, it is 3.5 times as likely that CAD is present.
   3. The LR for a given test can be found in epidemiology textbooks or calculated using the formulas given in IV B 2.
      a. Most diagnostic tests have an LR in the 2–5 range for positive test results and in the 0.5–0.2 range for negative results. These types of tests are only very useful if the pretest probability of disease is in the middle of the scale (e.g., 30%–70%). At either end of the probability scale, these

diagnostic tests do not greatly change the probability of disease.

   b. Good tests have LR^+ of 10 or more and LR^- of 0.1 or less. These powerful diagnostic tests can help rule in or rule out a diagnosis across a broader range of pretest probabilities. Unfortunately, these types of tests are often expensive or invasive.

   c. In order to truly rule in or rule out disease across the full range of pretest probabilities, a test must have an LR^+ of 100 or more and an LR^- of 0.01 or less. Very few tests (e.g., cardiac catheterization) have likelihood ratios this high or this low.

C. The **posttest probability** is the probability that a specific disease is present after a diagnostic test. Once we have determined the **pretest probability** of disease (using clinical information and disease prevalence data) and the **LR** of the diagnostic test result, we are ready to calculate the **posttest probability**. First, however, the pretest probability must be converted to odds (the LR already is expressed in odds).

$$\text{Pretest probability} \rightarrow \text{Pretest odds} \times LR =$$
$$\text{Posttest odds} \rightarrow \text{Posttest probability}$$

1. Steps

   a. Pretest probability must be converted to pretest odds:

$$\text{Odds} = \frac{(\text{Probability})}{(1 - \text{Probability})}$$

(For example, a probability of 75% equals an odds of 3:1).

   b. Pretest odds are multiplied by the LR to give posttest odds.

   c. Posttest odds must then be converted back to posttest probability:

$$\text{Probability} = \frac{(\text{Odds})}{(\text{Odds} + 1)}$$

2. Examples

   a. In the 45-year-old man with the atypical chest pain and a positive treadmill test, the posttest probability of disease would be 78%:

     (1) The 50% pretest probability is converted to pretest odds: $(0.5)/(1 - 0.5) = (0.5)/(0.5) = 1:1$.

     (2) The 1:1 pretest odds are multiplied by the LR (3.5) to yield posttest odds of 3.5:1.

      (3) The posttest odds are converted to a posttest probability: $(3.5)/(3.5 + 1) = (3.5)/(4.5) = 0.78$ or 78%.

   b. In the 30-year-old woman with atypical chest pain and a positive treadmill test, the posttest probability would be 16%.

   c. In the 60-year-old man with typical angina and a positive treadmill test, the posttest probability would be 98.5%.

 3. In order to gain diagnostic strength, several tests may be combined, as long as they are independent tests;

$$\textbf{Pretest odds} \times \textbf{LR}_1 \times \textbf{LR}_2 \times \textbf{LR}_3 = \textbf{Posttest odds}$$

where LR_1 is the likelihood ratio of the first test, LR_2 is the likelihood ratio of the second test, and LR_3 is the likelihood ratio of the third test.

References

Chou TM, Amidon TM: Evaluating coronary artery disease noninvasively-which test for whom? *West J Med* 161:173–180, 1994.

Sackett DL, Haynes RB, Tugwell P: *Clinical Epidemiology: A Basic Science for Clinical Medicine.* Boston, Little, Brown, 1985.

Sackett DL, Richardson WS, Rosenberg W, Haynes RB: *Evidence-Based Medicine: How to Practice and Teach EBM.* New York, Churchill Livingstone, 1998.

4. Noninvasive Diagnostic Testing

....

I INTRODUCTION

A. Noninvasive diagnostic tests are invaluable in the assessment of patients with suspected cardiac disease.

B. The judicious use of noninvasive diagnostic tests can help the clinician screen for disease, make an accurate diagnosis, and guide therapy while limiting the costs, risks, and discomfort associated with more invasive tests.

II ELECTROCARDIOGRAM (ECG)

A. Purpose. The ECG is an inexpensive, noninvasive, and widely available test that rapidly provides valuable information regarding cardiac structure and function. It is often the first diagnostic test performed in the cardiac evaluation of a patient.

B. Interpretation. See Chapter 2 for a discussion on ECG interpretation.

III CHEST ROENTGENOGRAM

A. Purpose. The chest radiograph can provide important information regarding cardiac structure and function.

B. Interpretation. Reading the chest film using an "outside-in" approach ensures that commonly overlooked structures (e.g., bones) are not forgotten.

   1. Bones

      a. Rib notching indicates coarctation of the aorta (see Chapter 25, Figure 25-1).

      b. Lytic or blastic lesions may signal a metastatic malignancy, which may be associated with a pericardial effusion.

   2. Lungs. Examining the parenchyma and vasculature of the lungs can provide important clues to the presence of heart disease.

      a. Congestive heart failure (CHF) may be suspected if pulmonary edema or **cephalization** is present. Cephalization is the redistribution of blood flow toward the apices and is characterized by dilatation of the upper pulmonary vessels and constriction of the lower pulmonary vessels (see Chapter 16, Figure 16-2).

b. Pulmonary hypertension may be suspected if the central pulmonary arteries are dilated (greater than the size of a dime), with pruning of the peripheral branches.

3. Heart

  a. Cardiomegaly. The cardiac silhouette should be less than one-half of the thoracic diameter on a posterior–anterior (PA) film; anything larger indicates cardiomegaly.

HOT

KEY

A "globular" shape to the heart with normal pulmonary vasculature may indicate a pericardial effusion (see Chapter 21, Figure 21-2).

---

  b. Chamber enlargement

  (1) The left side of the cardiac silhouette represents the left ventricle, whereas the right side represents the right atrium. Prominence in either location may indicate enlargement of the respective chamber.

  (2) Left atrial enlargement may be signified by:

  (a) The loss of the normal concavity on the left side of the heart

  (b) An elevated left mainstem bronchus

  (c) The "**double-density**" **sign,** which is seen as two parallel lines on the right side of the heart representing the right atrial and the enlarged left atrial borders

  (3) Right ventricular enlargement is best seen on a lateral film as filling of the retrosternal space.

4. Mediastinum

  a. Mediastinal widening may signify aortic dissection or aneurysm.

  b. The **"figure 3" sign** may be seen with coarctation of the aorta (see Chapter 25, Figure 25-1). The three parts of the sign represent:

  (1) The dilated aorta above the coarctation

  (2) The central indentation from the coarctation itself

  (3) The poststenotic dilatation just below the coarctation

IV TESTS FOR ARRHYTHMIAS

A. The **ambulatory ECG monitor** (i.e., Holter monitor) is used for patients with suspected arrhythmias or myocardial ischemia.

  1. Methodology

  a. The patient wears a small portable box that is connected to three ECG leads. The box continuously records the patient's heart rhythm over a 24- to 48-hour period.

     b. The patient also keeps a **diary,** which allows correlation between symptoms and arrhythmias.

  2. Clinical applications

     a. The Holter monitor can be used to record the initiation, rate, and duration of:

       (1) Bradyarrhythmias [e.g., sinus node dysfunction, atrioventricular (AV) block]

       (2) Tachyarrhythmias (e.g., supraventricular tachycardia, ventricular tachycardia)

     b. The Holter monitor also can be used to detect the number and total duration of **ischemic episodes**. Holter monitoring of ST-segment depression may be useful in diagnosing patients with suspected coronary artery disease (CAD), as well as following a patient's response to antianginal therapy.

B. An **event monitor** is very similar to a Holter monitor, but the patient wears the device for a longer period (1–3 months).

  1. Methodology. Upon feeling symptoms (e.g., palpitations, lightheadedness), the patient must manually activate the event monitor by hitting the record button on the box. With each activation, the event monitor will save the ECG rhythm for several minutes before and after the episode.

  2. Clinical applications. The event monitor is useful for patients who experience infrequent symptoms suggestive of arrhythmias. Because of the infrequency of the arrhythmias, the Holter monitor may not detect them during the 24- to 48-hour recording.

C. The **signal-averaged ECG (SAECG)** is a noninvasive test that can stratify a patient's risk of developing life-threatening ventricular arrhythmias.

  1. Methodology

     a. The SAECG is performed using the standard ECG leads. The patient's risk potential is calculated by averaging the data from approximately 200 QRS complexes.

     b. The SAECG displays waveforms (i.e., **late potentials**) within the terminal portion of the QRS complex and ST segments that have too low an amplitude and too high a frequency for the standard ECG equipment to detect.

  2. Clinical applications

     a. While a normal SAECG identifies a patient at low risk for arrhythmias, an abnormal SAECG is not highly accurate in predicting future adverse arrhythmias.

     b. Abnormal late potentials are associated with an approximate six-fold increase in arrhythmic events and are more common in patients with prior myocardial infarction (MI).

    c. In patients with prior MI and a depressed left ventricular ejection fraction (LVEF), the SAECG may be useful for identifying those at high risk for serious ventricular arrhythmias. These patients may require invasive electrophysiologic testing (see Chapter 5).

D. The **tilt table test** is used in the workup of patients suspected of having recurrent vasovagal syncope.

    1. Methodology

       a. The patient is placed on a table, and the heart rate and blood pressure are recorded. Then the table is tilted upright 60°–80° for 30 minutes.

       b. If no bradycardia or hypotension is detected, the test can be repeated using provocation with carotid sinus massage or intravenous isoproterenol.

    2. Clinical applications

       a. The **test is positive** if the patient experiences symptoms (e.g., lightheadedness, loss of consciousness) accompanied by a drop in heart rate and blood pressure.

       b. If the tilt table test is positive, the diagnosis of vasovagal syncope is supported.

V TESTS FOR CARDIAC STRUCTURE AND FUNCTION

A. Echocardiography is a diagnostic test that uses ultrasound imaging to evaluate the structure and function of the heart.

    1. Imaging approaches

       a. Transthoracic echocardiography (TTE) is a noninvasive approach. A hand-held ultrasound probe is placed over the chest wall and the images are obtained through the chest wall.

       b. Transesophageal echocardiography (TEE) is a more invasive approach. After being intravenously sedated, the patient swallows a long steerable tube with the ultrasound probe on its tip. Clinical applications include:

          (1) Imaging from inside the esophagus and stomach allows a much clearer view of the cardiac structures compared with imaging through the chest wall.

          (2) TEE is superior to TTE for the diagnosis of aortic dissection, endocarditis, thrombi, and masses.

    2. Modes of imaging

       a. Two-dimensional echocardiography (2DE)

          (1) Methodology. 2DE is an imaging mode that displays a wedge-shaped sector of the heart (Figure 4-1). The image is obtained by using a variety of standard views, which provide different "slices" through the heart.

          (2) Clinical applications. 2DE provides important information regarding the following:

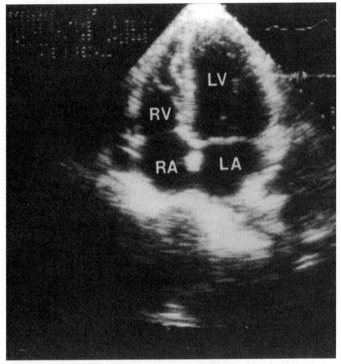

FIGURE 4-1. Normal view of the four chambers of the heart from a two-dimensional transthoracic echocardiogram. (Courtesy of N.B. Schiller, M.D., San Francisco, CA) *LA* = left atrium; *LV* = left ventricle; *RA* = right atrium; *RV* = right ventricle.

   (a) The size of the heart chambers
   (b) The ventricular ejection fraction (which can be calculated using the following equation):

$$\frac{\text{(end-diastolic volume)} - \text{(end-systolic volume)}}{\text{(end-diastolic volume)}}$$

   (c) The structure of the valves
   (d) The appearance of the pericardium
b. M-mode echocardiography
   (1) Methodology. M-mode echocardiography is produced by sweeping the ultrasound probe through one plane and plotting the image depth against time (Figure 4-2).
   (2) Clinical applications. M-mode echocardiography is particularly useful for calculating ventricular size and systolic function, as well as for looking at mitral and

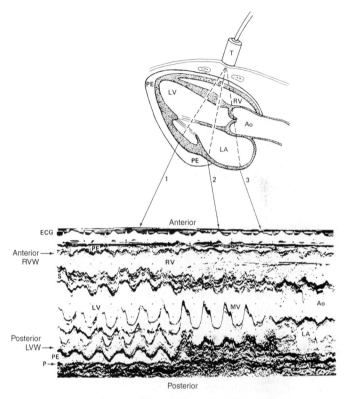

FIGURE 4-2. In M-mode echocardiography, the normal intracardiac structures can be seen by moving the transducer from position 1 to position 3. In this case, a small pericardial effusion can also be seen. (Courtesy of N.B. Schiller, M.D., San Francisco, CA) *Ao* = aorta; *ECG* = electrocardiogram; *LA* = left atrium; *LV* = left ventricle; *LVW* = left ventricular wall; *MV* = mitral valve; *PE* = pericardial effusion; *P* = pericardium; *RV* = right ventricle; *RVW* = right ventricular wall; *T* = transducer.

aortic leaflet motion to detect valvular stenosis, prolapse, or rupture.

   c. **Doppler echocardiography** provides information regarding the flow of blood through the heart.

      (1) **Color flow Doppler** provides shades of color to represent the speed and direction of blood movement. This type of imaging is useful in assessing regurgitant valve lesions and intracardiac shunts [e.g., ventricular septal defect (VSD)].

      (2) **Spectral Doppler** can quantitatively measure blood flow indices, allowing for assessment of stroke vol-

ume, pulmonary artery pressure, and the severity of aortic regurgitation and valvular stenosis.

B. Nuclear cardiology has developed tests of left and right ventricular function. **Radionuclide angiocardiography** is useful for testing ventricular function and involves mixing a radioactive tracer in the blood and measuring the counts arising from the heart chamber (which are proportional to chamber volume). Two principal methods can be used:

1. The **first pass method** records the initial circulation of the radionuclide through the blood.

2. The gated method, also referred to as **multiple gated acquisition (MUGA),** records the circulation of the radionuclide through multiple cardiac cycles and records the images at different points in time during the cycle. This method allows an accurate, safe, and highly reproducible measurement of the left and right ventricular ejection fractions.

C. Ultrafast computed tomography (CT) is a new technology that allows imaging of the cardiovascular system.

1. **Methodology.** CT images are obtained while the patient holds his breath to minimize motion artifact.

2. **Clinical applications**

   a. Currently, ultrafast CT is best suited for imaging of aortic dissections and aneurysms, pericardial calcification and effusion, and intracardiac tumors (e.g., atrial myxoma, cardiac metastasis).

   b. If ultrafast CT detects coronary artery calcification, CAD may be suspected. The accuracy of this diagnosis, however, remains controversial.

   c. The clinical utility of ultrafast CT is promising; however, further investigation is needed.

D. Magnetic resonance imaging (MRI)

1. **Methodology.** MRI is a noninvasive, but expensive, imaging modality.

2. **Clinical applications**

   a. MRI provides remarkably clear images of the heart chambers, thus allowing for:

      (1) Estimation of ventricular hypertrophy

      (2) Assessment of ventricular function

      (3) Identification of cardiac masses and thrombi

      (4) Diagnosis of aortic dissections or aneurysms

   b. Currently, the use of MRI is limited largely because of its cost.

VI TESTS FOR CORONARY ARTERY DISEASE (CAD) are useful for diagnosing CAD, assessing its severity, and evaluating a patient's prognosis.

A. The **treadmill exercise test** is the most widely used screening test for CAD.

   1. Methodology

      a. The patient walks on an inclined treadmill, gradually increasing its speed and incline. During the exercise, the patient's symptoms (e.g., dyspnea, chest pain, lightheadedness), 12-lead ECG, and blood pressure are closely monitored.

      b. The most common exercise treadmill test is the **Bruce protocol.** This procedure is divided into seven 3-minute stages, and both the speed and the incline of the treadmill are increased with each stage.

HOT

KEY

Typically, the heart rate goal during an exercise test is 85% of the patient's maximum predicted heart rate (MPHR), which can be calculated by subtracting the patient's age from 220. Attaining a "submaximal" heart rate (less than 85% of the MPHR) during the test may not induce the electrocardiographic abnormalities indicative of ischemia in patients with CAD.

---

   2. Abnormal responses to exercise testing

      a. ST segment depression

         (1) The presence of 1 mm of down-sloping or horizontal ST segment depression, or 2 mm of up-sloping ST segment depression indicates exercise-induced myocardial ischemia.

         (2) If abnormal ST segment depression develops within 3 minutes of the start of exercise, the patient should be further evaluated for left main or three-vessel CAD.

      b. Hypotension (systolic pressure falls more than 10 mm Hg) is an infrequent, ominous finding that suggests severe CAD with left ventricular systolic dysfunction.

      c. Ventricular arrhythmias, during or after exercise, may be a sign of severe CAD. Coronary angiography should be considered.

      d. Poor exercise tolerance (i.e., less than 6 minutes of exercise) is associated with a poor prognosis. However, patients who can exercise longer than 12 minutes (even if ischemia is present) have a good prognosis.

B. Myocardial perfusion scintigraphy

   1. Methodology. Myocardial perfusion scintigraphy often is performed in conjunction with the treadmill exercise test and involves the intravenous administration of thallium-201 or technetium-99m sestamibi.

      a. Myocardial perfusion scintigraphy is particularly useful in assessing patients with an uninterpretable baseline ECG [e.g., left bundle branch block (LBBB), ventricular pacing complexes, left ventricular hypertrophy (LVH) with repolarization abnormality, digoxin effect].

    b. Ventricular wall motion and perfusion are recorded at rest and compared with that recorded immediately after exercise.

  2. Clinical applications

    a. The administration of these radionuclides is useful because cardiac muscle cells that are ischemic or infarcted show a decrease in isotope uptake.

    b. Reversible defects, areas that lack isotope uptake on exercise images but "fill in" on resting images, indicate ischemia.

    c. Fixed defects, areas that show no change in isotope uptake on resting images, usually denote infarction.

C. Pharmacologic stress test. Patients who are unable to exercise on a treadmill (because of peripheral vascular, pulmonary, neurologic, or musculoskeletal diseases) may be evaluated using vasodilator agents (e.g., intravenous dipyridamole, adenosine, dobutamine) along with nuclear perfusion or echocardiographic imaging.

  1. Methodology

    a. Intravenous **dipyridamole** or **adenosine** produces a greater extent of vasodilation in normal coronary arteries compared with vasodilation in atherosclerotic vessels. This difference in vasodilation causes the isotope to shunt away from those cardiac regions served by diseased vessels. These agents are contraindicated in patients with active bronchospasm.

    b. Intravenous **dobutamine** increases oxygen demand by increasing heart rate and contractility, and may be used as an alternative to exercise in stress echocardiographic studies.

  2. Clinical applications. If exercise or pharmacologic stress results in a decrease in the LVEF or segmental wall motion abnormalities, cardiac ischemia may be presumed.

HOT **KEY** If during exercise the echocardiogram shows the development of mitral regurgitation, ischemia of the mitral papillary muscle resulting from right or left circumflex CAD may be present. Ischemic mitral regurgitation should be suspected in patients who present with acute pulmonary edema.

References
Fletcher GF, Schlant RC: The Exercise Test. In *Hurst's The Heart,* 9th ed. Edited by Alexander RW, Schlant RC, Fuller V. New York, McGraw-Hill, 1998, pp 519–536.

5. Invasive Diagnostic Testing

I   INTRODUCTION

A. Invasive diagnostic testing can help the clinician obtain a definitive assessment, determine important prognostic information, and guide therapy.

   1. Cardiac catheterization and coronary angiography are used in the assessment of myocardial, valvular, and coronary artery disorders.

   2. Electrophysiologic studies (EPS) are used in the workup of patients with possible arrhythmias. The results of EPS are helpful not only for accurately diagnosing the arrhythmia, but also for guiding antiarrhythmic therapy.

B. Before proceeding with an invasive diagnostic test, the risks of the procedure [e.g., myocardial infarction (MI), stroke, arrhythmia, infection, death] must be weighed against the benefits of testing.

II   RIGHT HEART CATHETERIZATION

A. Methodology. Right heart catheterization (RHC) is performed by introducing a Swan-Ganz pulmonary artery catheter through a large vein (e.g., femoral, internal jugular, or subclavian vein). The catheter is then guided to the right atrium, then across the tricuspid valve to the right ventricle, and finally across the pulmonic valve to the pulmonary artery.

B. Indications for use. RHC may be considered in patients with shock, congestive heart failure (CHF), suspected intracardiac shunt, and pulmonary hypertension.

C. Hemodynamic measurements

   1. Right heart pressure (Figure 5-1). Pressure tracings can be recorded from the right atrium, right ventricle, pulmonary artery, and pulmonary capillary wedge (PCW) positions (see Appendix A for normal values).

   2. Cardiac output (CO) is the quantity of blood delivered into the systemic circulation; it is usually expressed in liters per minute (L/min). CO can be determined by two methods, each of which requires proper placement of the Swan-Ganz catheter.

   a. Thermodilution method

   (1) Technique. Ten milliliters of cold saline are injected into the proximal right atrial port of the Swan-Ganz catheter. A thermistor at the distal tip of the catheter

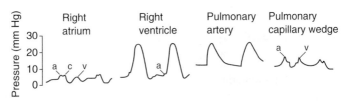

FIGURE 5-1. Normal heart pressures obtained with a Swan-Ganz catheter.

in the pulmonary artery detects the speed at which the cool saline reaches the pulmonary artery, thus calculating the CO.

(2) **Limitations.** This method is not always accurate for patients with significant tricuspid regurgitation or very low CO states.

b. **Fick method.** In most cases, this technique overcomes the limitations associated with the thermodilution method.

(1) **Overview**

(a) Pulmonary blood flow (which is equal to systemic blood flow) is determined by calculating the difference in oxygen content between the oxygenated arterial blood and the deoxygenated venous blood.

(b) As the CO drops, the venous blood will have a lower oxygen content because the peripheral tissues are extracting more oxygen.

(2) **Technique.** The Fick method uses the following equation to calculate CO:

$$CO = \text{(Oxygen consumption)} / \text{(Arteriovenous oxygen difference)}$$

(a) **Oxygen consumption** is the rate at which the body uses oxygen; it is usually expressed in milliliters of oxygen per minute (ml/min). The oxygen consumption can be estimated as 3 ml/min/kg, or more definitively determined by using a Douglas bag, which measures the oxygen content in the patient's expired air.

(b) **The arteriovenous oxygen difference** can be calculated using the following equation:

$$\text{Arteriovenous oxygen difference} = (13.9)\,(SaO_2 - SvO_2)\,(Hb),$$

where

SaO_2 = the oxygen saturation in arterial blood

SvO_2 = the oxygen saturation in venous blood, usually taken from the pulmonary artery

Hb = hemoglobin (g/dl)

(3) Limitations. The Fick method requires that there is no intracardiac shunt (e.g., atrial or ventricular septal defect) so that the pulmonary blood flow is equal to the systemic blood flow.

3. Intracardiac shunts

a. Cardiac catheterization can be used to detect, localize, and quantify intracardiac shunts by documenting changes in the oxygen saturation. The **oximetry run** is the technique used to document changes in oxygen saturation.

   (1) Oxygen saturation typically is measured in the inferior and superior vena cavae, the right atrium, the right ventricle, and the pulmonary artery.

   (2) An increase (termed "step-up") in the oxygen saturation value of 8% or more may represent a left-to-right intracardiac shunt.

b. Ventricular septal defect (VSD)

   (1) A left-to-right shunt at the ventricular level will show an increase in oxygen saturation from the right atrium to the right ventricle.

   (2) The flow ratio of pulmonary blood (Qp) to systemic blood (Qs) is a useful measure of the size of an intracardiac shunt. A simplified formula for the Qp/Qs ratio in a patient with a VSD is:

$$[(SaO_2 - SvO_2)]/[(SpvO_2 - SpaO_2)],$$

where

SaO_2 = the oxygen saturation in the arterial blood

SvO_2 = the mixed venous oxygen saturation from the right atrium

$SpvO_2$ = the oxygen saturation of the pulmonary vein

$SpaO_2$ = the oxygen saturation of the pulmonary artery

c. Atrial septal defect (ASD)

   (1) A left-to-right shunt at the atrial level will show an increase in oxygen saturation from the vena cavae to the right atrium.

   (2) The equation for calculating the flow ratio of pulmonary blood to systemic blood (Qp/Qs) in a patient with an ASD is similar to the equation given for a VSD, except the SvO_2 is the mixed venous oxygen saturation from the vena cavae. The mixed venous oxygen saturation is calculated from the superior vena cava (SVC) and inferior vena cava (IVC) using the following equation:

$$[3(SVC) + 1(IVC)] / 4$$

D. Risks. In general, the risks of RHC are minor with complications resulting from:
   1. Venous sheath insertion, which can lead to pneumothorax, hemothorax, or hematoma
   2. Arrhythmias (e.g., supraventricular and ventricular)

HOT

▶

KEY

Insertion of the Swan-Ganz catheter can cause transient right bundle branch block (RBBB) in some patients. For patients with a preexisting left bundle branch block (LBBB), placement of a temporary transvenous pacemaker is usually recommended prior to Swan-Ganz catheter placement to prevent the possibility of complete heart block.

III LEFT HEART CATHETERIZATION AND CORONARY ANGIOGRAPHY

A. Methodology
   1. **LHC** involves advancing a catheter through a large artery (e.g., femoral, brachial, or radial artery) across the aortic valve and into the left ventricle.
   2. **Coronary angiography** involves selectively injecting contrast dye into the coronary arteries. It is considered the "gold-standard" test to document the presence of coronary artery disease (CAD).
      a. Technique
         (1) Specially shaped catheters are advanced into the femoral, brachial, or radial artery to selectively engage the left and right coronary ostia.
         (2) Contrast media is injected into the coronary arteries, and the images are recorded using 35-mm cineangiographic film or digital processing.
      b. Findings. The location and extent of atherosclerotic coronary disease, characteristics of coronary blood flow, and presence of collateral vessels can be determined.
      c. Provocative testing may be used in patients with suspected **variant** (or **Prinzmetal's**) **angina.**
         (1) The test is positive if angina occurs, angiographic evidence of vasospasm is demonstrated, or ST segment deviation on the electrocardiogram (ECG) develops,

following the intravenous administration of **er-gonovine**.

(2) Provocative testing should be avoided in patients with severe atherosclerotic disease due to high-grade stenoses.

3. **Ventriculography**

a. **Technique.** Typically, a pigtail catheter is advanced into the ventricle and approximately 30–60 ml of contrast is injected within 2–4 seconds.

b. **Findings**

(1) Ventriculography provides angiographic assessment of right or left ventricular size and systolic function.

(2) Regurgitant jets from tricuspid or mitral regurgitation may also be detected during right or left ventriculography, respectively.

B. **Indications for use**

1. LHC may be considered for patients with CHF, suspected aortic or mitral valvular disease, and congenital heart disease.

2. **Coronary angiography**

a. Coronary angiography may be considered for patients with **known or suspected CAD who are candidates for revascularization** with angioplasty or bypass surgery. Suitable candidates typically meet one or more of the following criteria:

(1) Stable or unstable angina refractory to medical therapy

(2) An early positive stress test that suggests left main or three-vessel coronary disease

(3) MI complicated by postinfarction angina, CHF, or an abnormal stress test

(4) Acute myocardial infarction (AMI) that occurs prior to a planned angioplasty or as a result of failed thrombolytic therapy

(5) An abnormal stress test in patients scheduled for noncardiac surgery (see Chapter 30)

(6) Planned cardiovascular surgery (e.g., valve replacement, aortic aneurysm repair)

(7) Recurrent angina following angioplasty or bypass surgery, when restenosis or early graft failure is suspected

b. Coronary angiography may also be considered when CAD is suspected, but the diagnosis is unclear after noninvasive testing.

3. **Ventriculography** may be considered in patients with suspected left ventricular systolic dysfunction, mitral regurgitation, or VSD.

C. Hemodynamic measurements
   1. **Left heart pressure** (Figure 5-2) is measured from a catheter advanced across the aortic valve into the left ventricle.
   2. The **stenotic valve area** can be calculated using the **Hakki formula,** a simplified form of the Gorlin formula, which requires accurate pressure recordings and CO measurements:

$$\textbf{Valve area} = \textbf{CO} / \sqrt{\textbf{(Mean pressure gradient across the valve)}}$$

If the CO is high, the valve area is large. If the pressure gradient across the valve is high, the valve area is small.
   a. **Aortic stenosis**
      (1) The mean systolic pressure gradient is measured by simultaneously measuring the left ventricular and aortic pressures.
      (2) For example, if the CO is 5 L/min and the mean aortic valve pressure gradient is 40 mm Hg, the aortic valve area is 5 divided by the square root of 40, showing a valve area of 0.79 cm^2.
   b. **Mitral stenosis**
      (1) The left atrial pressure is estimated by measuring the PCW using a Swan-Ganz catheter. The mean diastolic pressure gradient is measured by simultaneously measuring the PCW and the left ventricular pressures.
      (2) For example, if the CO is 5 L/min, and the mean mitral valve pressure gradient is 30 mm Hg, the mitral valve area is 0.91 cm^2.
D. Risks. The risks associated with LHC, coronary angiography, and ventriculography range from minor transient problems (e.g., bradycardia during coronary contrast injection) to major complications (Table 5-1). The overall risk of a major complication, however, is less than 1%.
   1. **Renal dysfunction**
      a. **Contrast-induced**

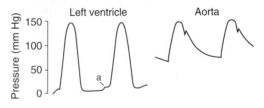

FIGURE 5-2. Normal left heart pressures obtained with a pigtail catheter.

TABLE 5-1. Major Complications of Cardiac Catheterization, Angiography, and Ventriculography

Complication	Incidence (%)
Death	0.1
Myocardial infarction	0.1
Stroke	0.1
Arrhythmias requiring countershock or temporary pacing	0.3
Local vascular disorder (e.g., retroperitoneal bleeding, hematoma, vessel thrombosis, false aneurysm formation, distal embolization)	1.5
Vasovagal reaction	2
Renal dysfunction	1–5
Contrast reaction	2

(1) **Mechanism.** Renal dysfunction, as a result of contrast administration, is caused by 2 mechanisms:
   (a) The contrast is directly toxic to the renal tubules.
   (b) The contrast causes vasoconstriction of the renal arteries (resulting in a prerenal state).
(2) **Incidence**. A rise in the serum creatinine level by 1 mg/dl or more may occur in as many as 5% of patients. Less than 1% of patients, however, develop renal dysfunction requiring chronic dialysis.
(3) **Risk factors**. Contrast-induced renal dysfunction occurs more frequently in patients with preexisting renal dysfunction, diabetes, multiple myeloma, and dehydration. Patients receiving nephrotoxic medication may also be at risk.
(4) **Clinical characteristics.** The elevation in serum creatinine usually peaks 1–2 days after cardiac catheterization and may return to baseline within 1 week.
(5) **Preventive measures.** For patients with an increased risk for renal dysfunction, preventive measures include:
   (a) The intravenous administration of 0.5% normal saline for 12 hours before and after the procedure
   (b) Minimization of the amount of contrast used
b. **Systemic cholesterol embolization**
(1) **Mechanism.** Cholesterol emboli, migrating from the aorta to the renal arteries, often damage the renal tubules. Renal failure develops slowly over weeks to months.
(2) **Incidence.** Systemic cholesterol embolization may occur in approximately 0.1% of patients.

      (3) Risk factors. Systemic cholesterol embolization is more common in patients with diffuse atherosclerosis, particularly those with extensive aortic plaque.

      (4) Clinical characteristics. Systemic cholesterol embolization may result in:

         (a) Livido reticularis, a persistent rash, characterized by a symmetric, bluish, mesh-like pattern on the extremities and occasionally the trunk

         (b) Abdominal or foot pain

         (c) Systemic eosinophilia

         (d) Cholesterol clefts on renal biopsy

      (5) Preventive measures. Heparinization and careful technique while manipulating the catheters in the aorta may decrease the risk of plaque embolization.

2. Contrast reaction

    a. Mechanism. Contrast activates the complement cascade, resulting in histamine release from circulating basophil and tissue mast cells.

    b. Incidence

      (1) Allergic reactions (e.g., hives) occur in 2% of cases.

      (2) Anaphylactoid reactions (e.g., hypotension, airway edema) occur in 0.1% of cases.

    c. Risk factors. Patients with a known iodine, contrast, or shellfish allergy are at an increased risk for a contrast reaction.

    d. Clinical characteristics. The release of histamine may cause urticaria, angioedema of the lips and eyelids, bronchospasm, or hypotension.

    e. Preventive measures. For a patient with a well-documented severe contrast reaction, the clinician should use non-ionic contrast and administer the following agents for 24–48 hours prior to and following cardiac catheterization:

      (1) Prednisone, 20 mg orally, three times a day

      (2) H_1 blocker (e.g., diphenhydramine), 25 mg orally, three times a day

      (3) H_2 blocker (e.g., ranitidine), 150 mg orally, two times a day

---

HOT KEY

The oral hypoglycemic agent metformin (Glucophage) should not be administered within 48 hours prior to or following cardiac catheterization because of the risk of contrast-related metabolic acidosis and renal dysfunction. Of patients who develop these complications, there is a roughly 50% mortality rate.

IV **ELECTROPHYSIOLOGIC STUDIES** may be considered for patients with suspected arrhythmias when a noninvasive workup [i.e., electrocardiography, Holter monitoring, and echocardiography] fails to provide a clear diagnosis.

A. Methodology. EPS are performed in the cardiac catheterization laboratory by cardiac electrophysiologists. Electrode catheters are advanced from the femoral or internal jugular veins to the right atrium, right ventricle, coronary sinus, and occasionally left atrium. These electrodes record electrical activity from different regions of the heart.

B. Indications for use. EPS are generally indicated for the following clinical situations:

1. **Suspected sinus or atrioventricular (AV) node dysfunction** in patients with syncope
2. **Narrow QRS complex tachycardia** in patients with frequent or poorly tolerated symptoms
3. **Wide QRS complex tachycardia** when the diagnosis of supraventricular versus ventricular tachycardia is unclear
4. **Suspected ventricular tachycardia** in patients who have survived a cardiac arrest

C. Goals. The goals of EPS include:

1. Assessment of the conduction system of the heart
2. Study of brady- and tachyarrhythmias
3. Determination of specific treatment, for example:
   a. Patients with inducible ventricular tachycardia (e.g., ventricular tachycardia triggered by pacing beats from a catheter) may be treated with antiarrhythmic medication or an automatic implantable defibrillator.
   b. Patients with either supraventricular or ventricular tachycardia may benefit from mapping of the tachycardia to help guide catheter or surgical ablation.
   c. Patients with Wolff-Parkinson-White syndrome, atrioventricular nodal reentry tachycardia (AVNRT) or atrial flutter are most effectively treated with catheter ablation (see Chapter 7).

References

Baim DS, Grossman W: *Cardiac Catheterization, Angiography, and Intervention,* 5th ed. Philadelphia, Williams & Wilkins, 1996.

Franch RH, Douglas JS, King SB: Cardiac catheterization and coronary arteriography. In *Hurst's the Heart,* 9th ed. Edited by Alexander RW, Schlant RC, Fuster V. New York, McGraw- Hill, 1998, pp 537–574.

PART II

ARRHYTHMIAS

6. Syncope

I INTRODUCTION

A. Definition. Syncope is a transient loss of consciousness and postural tone that is caused by inadequate cerebral blood flow.

B. Epidemiology. Syncope is extremely common, accounting for approximately 5% of medical admissions and 3% of emergency room visits. The lifetime incidence approaches 50% in some patient groups.

II CAUSES OF SYNCOPE.

The etiologies of syncope can be classified as cardiac, noncardiac, or unexplained. Because the prognosis is significantly worse for patients with cardiac syncope, it is important to determine the etiology of syncope.

A. Cardiac syncope
  1. Obstructive disorders
   a. The **flow of blood out of the left side of the heart** can be obstructed by aortic stenosis, hypertrophic cardiomyopathy, left atrial myxoma, and mitral stenosis.
   b. The **flow of blood to the lungs** can be obstructed by pulmonic valve stenosis, pulmonary hypertension, pulmonary embolism, and right atrial myxoma.
   c. The **filling of the right atrium** can be obstructed by cardiac tamponade.
   d. The **flow of blood to the vital organs** can be obstructed by aortic dissection.
  2. Ischemic disorders. Pump failure or arrhythmias may result from myocardial ischemia or infarction.
  3. Arrhythmic disorders
   a. Bradyarrhythmias [e.g., sinus bradycardia, sick sinus syndrome, second- and third-degree atrioventricular (AV) block] can interfere with cardiac output (CO). Carotid sinus hypersensitivity may result in bradycardia.
   b. Tachyarrhythmias (e.g., ventricular tachycardia, supraventricular tachycardia) can also cause syncope. Medications,

such as quinidine, may cause syncope due to polymorphic ventricular tachycardia (i.e., torsade de pointes).

B. Noncardiac syncope

1. **Vasovagal syncope,** also known as the "common faint" or neurally mediated or neurocardiogenic syncope, is the most common cause of syncope in young patients. It frequently is preceded by a painful or emotional stimulus.

2. **Situational** causes of syncope include micturition, defecation, swallowing, coughing, and exerting of the arm muscles (leading to subclavian steal).

3. **Orthostatic hypotension** can cause syncope.

4. **Neurogenic** causes of syncope include:

   a. **Autonomic insufficiency,** which is common in the elderly and in patients with diabetes

   b. **Transient ischemic attacks (TIAs),** which are extremely rare causes of syncope because the vertebrobasilar circulation must be involved

5. **Certain medications** (e.g., vasodilators, hypnotics, sedatives, nitrates, diuretics, α blockers) and **drug abuse** (e.g., cocaine, heroin, hypnotics, sedatives, alcohol) also can induce syncope.

6. **Psychogenic** syncope is a diagnosis of exclusion.

C. Unexplained syncope. As many as 50% of patients have unexplained syncope. After cardiac causes are excluded, a patient with this type of syncope has an excellent prognosis.

III APPROACH TO THE PATIENT. The evaluation of a patient with syncope must be approached in a rigorous, stepwise fashion to avoid missing life-threatening disease.

A. History and physical examination. A thorough history and physical examination is a very important aspect of the evaluation and may establish the diagnosis in many patients.

1. **Cardiac syncope.** A cardiac cause is more likely if the patient has any history suggestive of cardiac disease. In addition, findings on the physical examination may indicate a possible cardiac etiology of syncope.

   a. Lightheadedness during exercise, which may suggest an obstructive or arrhythmic disorder

   b. Physical findings of aortic stenosis or hypertrophic cardiomyopathy

   c. Angina, which suggests cardiac ischemia

   d. Palpitations, which may indicate an arrhythmic disorder

   e. A syncopal episode following manipulation of the neck, which suggests carotid sinus hypersensitivity

   f. Significant trauma following syncope, which suggests sudden and complete loss of consciousness and may indicate an arrhythmic disorder

2. **Noncardiac syncope**
   a. **Vasovagal.** Determine if the syncopal episode was preceded by a painful or emotional stimulus.
   b. **Situational.** Determine if the syncopal episode was preceded by micturition, defecation, swallowing, coughing, or exerting of the arm muscles.
   c. **Orthostatic hypotension.** Note if the patient reports light-headedness when "getting up quickly." Always check orthostatic vital signs in patients with syncope.
   d. **Neurogenic.** Determine if anyone witnessed convulsions, bowel or bladder incontinence, or other signs suggestive of a post-ictal state.

HOT KEY Although a seizure is not syncope, it can result in a loss of consciousness and, therefore, must be considered in the differential diagnosis.

   e. **Medications and drug abuse.** Determine which prescription or over-the-counter medications the patient is taking. Also, ask if the patient is abusing any illicit drugs.
   f. **Psychogenic.** A psychogenic cause of syncope (e.g., hyperventilation) should be considered after all other causes have been excluded.
B. **Electrocardiogram (ECG).** All patients with syncope should have an ECG, although this test can identify fewer than 10% of the causes of syncope. Look for evidence of acute or remote myocardial infarction (MI), left ventricular hypertrophy (LVH), arrhythmias, conduction system disease, and preexcitation syndromes.
C. **Risk assessment.** Patients should be separated into two groups: those without evidence of heart disease, and those who may have heart disease.
   1. **No evidence of heart disease.** Patients who meet all of the following criteria after a thorough history, physical examination, and ECG are at low risk for a cardiac cause, and additional cardiac testing may not be indicated:
      a. **Younger than 60 years old**
      b. **No evidence of coronary artery disease (CAD) or congestive heart failure (CHF)**
      c. **Normal ECG**
   2. **Possible heart disease.** Anyone who does not meet all the criteria in III C 1 is included in this group. If there is any suspicion of an obstructive, ischemic, or arrhythmic cause, admission and continuous ECG monitoring are indicated. Additional diagnostic tests need to be considered, including:

   a. Echocardiography, which allows assessment of valvular disease (e.g., aortic stenosis), ventricular hypertrophy (e.g., hypertrophic cardiomyopathy), and ventricular size and function
   b. Exercise treadmill testing, which can rule out exercise-induced myocardial ischemia
   c. Ambulatory ECG monitoring, which is widely used, but establishes a diagnosis in only a small percentage of patients (event or loop recorders may improve the diagnostic yield)
   d. Signal-averaged ECG (SAECG), which is considered a controversial test in patients with syncope
   e. Electrophysiologic testing, which is useful in patients at high risk for tachyarrhythmia (e.g., those with left ventricular dysfunction) or bradyarrhythmia (e.g., those with conduction disease on ECG), especially when a diagnosis cannot be established using noninvasive methods
   f. Tilt table testing, which can be useful for documenting vasovagal syncope; however, a positive test does not necessarily rule out other etiologies

IV **TREATMENT** is cause-specific.

A. Cardiac syncope. The treatment of any correctable cardiac abnormality should be the first consideration.
   1. Obstructive disorders
      a. Valvular stenosis. Consider surgical replacement or valvuloplasty for patients who have syncope as a result of aortic, mitral, or pulmonic stenosis.
      b. Hypertrophic cardiomyopathy. Administer β blockers or calcium channel blockers to alleviate the symptoms of hypertrophic cardiomyopathy. These patients should avoid vigorous physical exertion.
   2. Ischemic disorders. Treatment includes:
      a. The administration of antianginal medications (e.g., nitrates, β blockers, calcium channel blockers)
      b. Revascularization (e.g., angioplasty, coronary artery bypass surgery)
   3. Arrhythmic disorders
      a. Bradyarrhythmias
         (1) Patients generally require a permanent implantable pacemaker.
         (2) In some patients, however, the withdrawal or substitution of the medicine contributing to the bradycardia (e.g., β blocker, calcium channel blocker) may obviate the need for a pacemaker.
         (3) Patients with carotid sinus hypersensitivity generally

require a dual chamber pacemaker because pharmacologic treatment usually is unsuccessful.
  b. **Tachyarrhythmias**
    (1) **Supraventricular tachyarrhythmias**. Patients are generally treated with AV node blockers (e.g., β blockers, digoxin, calcium channel blockers), antiarrhythmic medications, or catheter ablation (see Chapter 7).
    (2) **Ventricular tachyarrhythmias**. Patients are generally treated with antiarrhythmic medications. Some patients also require an automatic implantable cardioverter-defibrillator (see Chapter 9).
B. Noncardiac syncope
  1. Vasovagal syncope
    a. General treatment for patients with recurrent vasovagal syncope includes administration of:
      (1) β Blockers with sympathomimetic activity (e.g., pindolol)
      (2) Anticholinergic agents (e.g., transdermal scopolamine)
    b. Patients with recurrent vasovagal syncope may benefit from fludrocortisone (0.1–1.0 mg/day) plus a high-salt diet.
    c. Patients with extreme cases of vasovagal syncope may require an AV sequential permanent pacemaker.
  2. Situational syncope
    a. To avoid syncope as a result of micturition, male patients should be advised to sit while urinating.
    b. To avoid postprandial syncope, patients should be instructed to:
      (1) Avoid taking hypotensive medications before meals
      (2) Rest in the supine position after meals
  3. Orthostatic hypotension. Treatment includes:
    a. Eliminating certain medications (e.g., antihypertensives, diuretics, antidepressants, phenothiazines)
    b. Administering fludrocortisone with a high-salt diet to increase intravascular volume for refractory cases

V PREVENTION

A. Medications and the use of alcohol or illicit drugs should be reviewed carefully.
B. Education about likely precipitants can help prevent recurrences.
C. For patients with chronic medical conditions [e.g., CHF, anemia, chronic obstructive pulmonary disease (COPD)], the syncope threshold may be decreased by optimizing the underlying chronic condition.

References

Farrehi PM, Santinga JT, Eagle KA: Syncope: diagnosis of cardiac and noncardiac causes. *Geriatrics* 50(11):24–30, 1995.

Henderson MC, Prabhu SD: Syncope: current diagnosis and treatment. *Curr Probl Cardiol* 22(5):242–296, 1997.

Kapoor WN: Workup and management of patients with syncope. *Med Clin North Am* 79(5):1153–1170, 1995.

Linzer M, Yang EH, Estes NA, et al: Diagnosing syncope. Part 1: Value of history, physical examination, and electrocardiography. Clinical Efficacy Assessment Project of the American College of Physicians. *Ann Inter Med* 126(12):989–996, 1997.

7. Narrow QRS Tachyarrhythmias

I **INTRODUCTION.** **Tachyarrhythmias** may pose a significant challenge in diagnosis and often are treated very differently. All tachyarrhythmias can be classified according to whether they are regular (same distance between successive QRS complexes) or irregular, and whether their QRS complex is narrow (< 0.12 second) or wide (≥ 0.12 second; see Chapter 9). Making these two determinations and consulting Table 7-1 can significantly narrow the diagnostic possibilities.

HOT **KEY**

All narrow, regular tachyarrhythmias are supraventricular, but the term supraventricular tachycardia (SVT) is classically used to refer to atrioventricular nodal reentrant tachycardia (AVNRT), atrioventricular reentrant tachycardia (AVRT), atrial tachycardia (AT), and atrial flutter.

II **NARROW, REGULAR TACHYARRHYTHMIAS**

A. **Differential diagnosis**
  1. **Sinus tachycardia**
     a. **Etiologies.** Sinus tachycardia is usually a physiologic response to **stress.** Important etiologies include:
        (1) **Low stroke volume states** from intravascular volume depletion
        (2) **Hypoxia** (e.g., from pulmonary embolus, pneumonia)
        (3) **Hypercatecholamine states** (e.g., from pain, anxiety, pheochromocytoma)
        (4) **Systemic factors** (e.g., fever, anemia, hyperthyroidism)
        (5) **Drugs** (e.g., β agonists, theophylline, caffeine, cocaine)
        (6) **Inappropriate sinus tachycardia,** although this is an etiology of exclusion
     b. **Electrocardiogram (ECG) appearance.** Upright P waves in leads I, II, and aVF are always followed by a QRS complex.

TABLE 7-1. Classification of Narrow QRS Tachyarrhythmias

Regular Rhythm	Irregular Rhythm
Sinus tachycardia	Atrial fibrillation
AVNRT	Atrial flutter with variable block
AVRT	Multifocal atrial tachycardia
AT	Frequent PACs
Atrial flutter	

AVNRT = atrioventricular nodal reentrant tachycardia; AVRT = atrioventricular reentrant tachycardia; AT = atrial tachycardia; PACs = premature atrial contractions.

HOT

▶

KEY

The maximum heart rate in sinus tachycardia = 220 minus the patient's age.

2. **AVNRT** accounts for more than 50% of all SVTs in adults.
   a. **Characteristics** include:
      (1) A heart rate of approximately 180 ± 20 beats/min
      (2) Isolated QRS complexes, pseudo S waves, or inverted P waves
      (3) Cannon *a* waves and a pounding sensation in the neck, noted during physical examination
   b. **Mechanism.** Many people have a dual atrioventricular (AV) node that contains a fast pathway with a long refractory period and a slow pathway with a short refractory period.
      (1) During **sinus rhythm,** the impulse is conducted down the fast pathway to the ventricles. Conduction down the fast pathway traverses the AV node retrograde and blocks the impulses on the slow pathway (Figure 7-1).
      (2) **Excitation loop.** A premature atrial contraction (PAC) may be blocked in the fast pathway secondary to its long refractory period. The impulse is then conducted down the slow pathway, which has a short refractory period. The impulse may then enter the fast pathway, which is no longer refractory, and activate the atria by retrograde conduction (Figure 7-2).
   c. **ECG appearance**
      (1) In **typical AVNRT** (90% of cases), a PAC begins the loop of excitation. The P wave is inverted and occurs

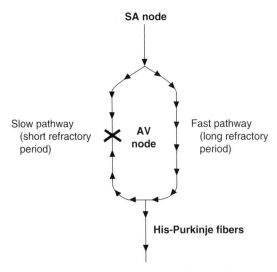

FIGURE 7-1. Dual atrioventricular node, sinus rhythm. *AV* = atrioventricular; *SA* = sinoatrial. (Reprinted with permission from Saint S, Frances C: *Saint-Frances Guide to Inpatient Medicine.* Philadelphia, Williams & Wilkins, 1997, p 36.)

          simultaneously with the QRS complex. **Only QRS complexes** are seen on the ECG.

    (2) In **atypical AVNRT** (10% of cases), a premature ventricular contraction (PVC) initiates the conduction of an impulse up the slow pathway and down the fast one (Figure 7-3). Because the retrograde P waves are formed from the slower pathway, they occur later and can be seen as **pseudo S waves** in the inferior leads (II, III, aVF) or as **inverted P waves** following the QRS complex.

3. AVRT accounts for more than 30% of all SVTs.

  a. Characteristics include a **short RP interval** on the ECG.

  b. Mechanism. AVRT involves an **accessory pathway,** which is an abnormal tract of fast conducting tissue between the atria and ventricles that bypasses the AV node. Accessory pathways often conduct in both an anterograde and retrograde direction.

  c. ECG appearance

    (1) Sinus rhythm

      (a) During sinus rhythm, anterograde conduction results in ventricular preexcitation, manifested as a

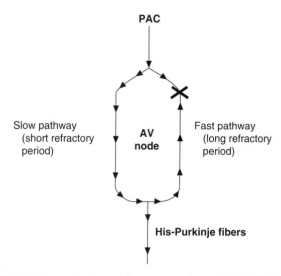

FIGURE 7-2. Atrioventricular nodal reentrant tachycardia (AVNRT) from premature atrial contractions (PACs). Following conduction down the slow pathway, the fast pathway is no longer refractory and may conduct retrograde, forming an excitation loop. *AV* = atrioventricular. (Reprinted with permission from Saint S, Frances C: *Saint-Frances Guide to Inpatient Medicine*. Philadelphia, Williams & Wilkins, 1997, p 37.)

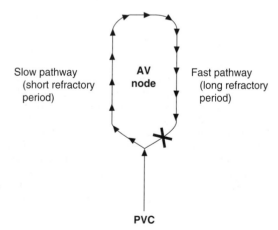

FIGURE 7-3. Atypical atrioventricular nodal reentrant tachycardia (AVNRT). *AV* = atrioventricular; *PVC* = premature ventricular contraction. (Reprinted with permission from Saint S, Frances C: *Saint-Frances Guide to Inpatient Medicine*. Philadelphia, Williams & Wilkins, 1997, p 38.)

short PR interval, prolongation of the QRS complex, and a **delta wave.**

   (b) If only retrograde conduction is possible (25% of cases), a **concealed bypass tract** is present and no abnormality is seen during sinus rhythm.

   (2) Excitation loop

   (a) **Orthodromic conduction** occurs when an impulse is conducted through the AV node and then up the accessory pathway in a retrograde direction (Figure 7-4). Because the loop is longer than that of AVNRT, the retrograde P wave is easily seen (i.e., it is not buried in the QRS complex). The interval from the QRS complex to the ensuing retrograde P wave is less than that from the P wave to the next QRS complex **(short RP or RP < PR tachycardia).** The QRS complex remains narrow because the ventricle is depolarized normally via the His-Purkinje system.

   (b) **Antidromic conduction** occurs when the impulse is conducted antegrade down the bypass tract. Antidromic conduction produces a **wide QRS complex** because the tract terminates in ventricular muscle fibers and conduction from myocardial fiber to fiber is slow.

4. AT accounts for 15% of all SVTs.

   a. Characteristics. The **atrial rate** is usually **less than 250 beats/min.**

   b. Mechanism. Enhanced automaticity of atrial tissue or atrial reentry is thought to be the mechanism.

   (1) Patients often have **structural heart disease.**

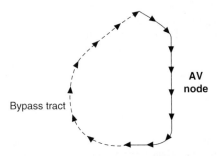

FIGURE 7-4. Orthodromic conduction leading to atrioventricular reentrant tachycardia (AVRT). *AV* = atrioventricular. (Reprinted with permission from Saint S, Frances C: *Saint-Frances Guide to Inpatient Medicine.* Philadelphia, Williams & Wilkins, 1997, p 39.)

(2) Because digoxin increases atrial and ventricular automaticity and depresses conduction in the AV node, AT with AV nodal block is a common presentation of **digoxin toxicity.**

  c. ECG appearance. A retrograde P wave, produced by depolarization low in the atria, is followed by a narrow QRS complex, generated by conduction of the impulse down the AV node. The preceding P wave is linked to the QRS complex, and the PR interval is shorter than the RP interval **(long RP** or **short PR tachycardia).**

HOT **KEY** The SVTs can be classified according to the RP interval:
      Short RP = AVRT and, occasionally, AVNRT
      Long RP = AT
      No RP = AVNRT

---

  5. Atrial flutter
    a. Characteristics
      (1) The atrial rate is often 300 beats/min, and the ventricular rate is approximately 150 beats/min with a 2:1 AV block.

HOT **KEY** Whenever the ventricular rate is 150 beats/min (±5), think of atrial flutter.

---

      (2) Atrial flutter is frequently transient and may degenerate to atrial fibrillation or return to sinus rhythm.
    b. Mechanism. Waves of organized depolarization move through the atria.
    c. ECG appearance. Because the waves often move in a superior-to-inferior direction, flutter waves are best seen in the inferior leads (i.e., leads II, III, and aVF).

B. Treatment
  1. Acute treatment depends on the patient's hemodynamic status.
    a. Hemodynamically unstable (or ischemic) patient
      (1) If the patient is **in sinus rhythm,** treat the underlying cause.
      (2) If the patient is **not in sinus rhythm,** initiate synchronized **electrical cardioversion** immediately.
    b. Hemodynamically stable patient
      (1) Carotid sinus massage may increase vagal tone and block impulses at the level of the AV node (Figure 7-5).

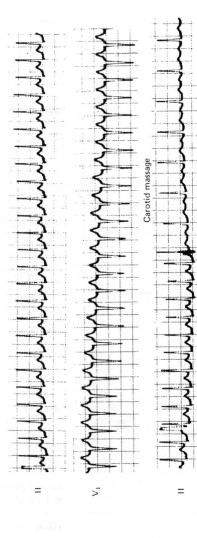

FIGURE 7-5. Carotid sinus massage led to the abrupt termination of a supraventricular tachycardia (SVT). (Reprinted with permission from Cheitlin MD, Sokolow M, McIlroy MB: *Clinical Cardiology*, 6th ed. Stamford, CT, Appleton & Lange, 1993, p 524).

Carotid sinus massage is contraindicated in the presence of a carotid bruit and should be performed with continuous ECG monitoring and a crash cart available.

- **(a) Sinus tachycardia.** Carotid sinus massage may slow the atrial rate.
- **(b) AVNRT** and **AVRT,** tachycardias that involve reentrant loops through the AV node, may terminate.
- **(c) AT** is usually unaffected by carotid sinus massage.
- **(d) Atrial flutter.** The flutter waves usually become more obvious as the AV block increases; the tachycardia will not terminate.

(2) If carotid sinus massage is ineffective, administer a rapid **intravenous bolus of adenosine** in incremental doses of 6 mg and then 12 mg. Halve the dose if administration is via a central line. The effects of adenosine occur within 15–30 seconds of administration and last for 10–20 seconds. Adenosine has effects similar to those of carotid sinus massage. Adenosine is contraindicated in patients with acute bronchospasm.

- **(a) Sinus tachycardia** transiently slows.
- **(b) AVNRT** and **AVRT.** More than 90% of these SVTs will terminate with a 12-mg dose.
- **(c) AT** rarely terminates. Intravenous administration of verapamil or diltiazem is preferable for arresting AT and may decrease the ventricular response, even if the tachycardia persists.
- **(d) Atrial flutter.** AV block increases and flutter waves are more evident. Additional treatment may involve AV nodal blockade with digoxin, β blockers, or calcium channel blockers, followed by either chemical (e.g., procainamide, sotalol, amiodarone propafenone, flecainide) or electrical cardioversion.

HOT KEY — In atrial flutter, antiarrhythmic class I_A agents (e.g., procainamide, quinidine) should not be given prior to the administration of AV nodal blocking agents. I_A drugs may increase AV nodal conduction sufficiently to permit 1:1 conduction through the AV node, thereby increasing the ventricular response.

---

2. Chronic treatment
- **a. AVNRT**
  - **(1)** Sporadic episodes may be controlled by vagal maneuvers.

    (2) For patients with frequent or serious episodes, AV nodal blocking agents or radiofrequency ablation (curative in 95% of cases) may be used.

b. AVRT

    (1) Symptomatic patients with evidence of preexcitation on a baseline ECG should probably be referred for radiofrequency ablation.

    (2) Symptomatic patients with no evidence of anterograde conduction (i.e., concealed bypass tract) can be treated with either ablation or an initial trial of an AV nodal blocking agent.

c. AT. Calcium channel blockers or β blockers are often the drugs of first choice. If pharmacologic therapy fails, ablation may be indicated. The success rate with ablation therapy, however, is much lower compared with the success rate for AVRT.

d. Atrial flutter usually degenerates to atrial fibrillation or reverts to sinus rhythm.

    (1) Typical atrial flutter has a roughly 90% cure rate with radiofrequency ablation.

    (2) Class I_A, I_C, or III antiarrhythmic medication often is useful for chronic rhythm control.

    (3) Anticoagulation strategies, similar to those used with atrial fibrillation, are recommended because of the risk of thromboembolism (see Chapter 8).

III NARROW, IRREGULAR TACHYARRHYTHMIAS

A. Differential diagnosis

1. Atrial fibrillation is discussed in detail in Chapter 8. This arrhythmia is characterized by irregular atrial fibrillatory waves at a rate of 350–600 beats/min and a ventricular rate of usually 120–160 beats/min.

2. Atrial flutter with variable block. To help differentiate atrial flutter with variable block from atrial fibrillation:

a. Look at the inferior leads (II, III, aVF). With atrial flutter, flutter waves can often be "marched out" at a rate of approximately 300 beats/min. Variable block will produce a ventricular rate in proportion to the atrial rate (i.e., the ventricular response to 2:1, 3:1, and 4:1 AV block will be 150 beats/min, 100 beats/min, and 75 beats/min, respectively).

b. Increase AV block by massaging the carotid sinus or administering intravenous adenosine. Flutter waves that may have been hidden will often become obvious when the ventricular response is slowed.

3. Multifocal atrial tachycardia (MAT)

a. Mechanism. In two-thirds of patients, MAT is associated with pulmonary disease. Cor pulmonale, for example, causes right atrial stretch, producing different foci of atrial contractions. Hypokalemia or hypomagnesemia may also cause MAT.

  b. ECG appearance. Diagnosis requires the presence of three distinct P wave morphologies and three different PR intervals in the same lead. As a result, the RR interval varies in an irregularly irregular pattern.

  4. Frequent PACs may give the appearance of an irregular rhythm.

B. Treatment

  1. Hemodynamically unstable (or ischemic) patients with **atrial fibrillation** or **atrial flutter with variable block** should undergo immediate **electrical cardioversion.** Cardioversion for patients with MAT is of no value.

  2. Hemodynamically stable patients

  a. Atrial fibrillation. Treatment is discussed in Chapter 8 VI.

  b. Atrial flutter with variable block. Treatment is the same as for atrial flutter without variable block (see section II B 1 b).

  c. MAT. The underlying condition (usually related to bronchospasm, hypoxia, hypercapnia, or metabolic derangements) should be treated. Intravenous verapamil often is tried, but this is a difficult arrhythmia to treat.

References

Basta M, Klein GJ, Yee R, et al: Current role of pharmacologic therapy for patients with paroxysmal supraventricular tachycardia. *Card Clin* 15(4):587–597, 1997.

Collier WW, Holt SE, Wellford LA: Narrow complex tachycardias. *Emerg Med Clin North Am* 13(4):925–954, 1995.

Fisch C: Electrocardiogram and mechanisms of arrhythmias. In *Cardiac Arrhythmia: Mechanisms, Diagnosis, and Management.* Edited by Podrid PJ, Kowey PR. Philadelphia, Williams & Wilkins, 1985, pp 211–218.

Ganz LI, Friedman PL: Supraventricular tachycardia. *N Engl J Med* 332(3):162–173, 1995.

8. Atrial Fibrillation

I INTRODUCTION

A. Epidemiology
1. Atrial fibrillation is the **most common chronic arrhythmia,** occurring in 2% of the general population. Of all hospitalized patients, 7% will have atrial fibrillation.
2. The **incidence varies with age:**
   a. Rare in people younger than 50 years
   b. One out of twenty people older than 60 years
   c. One out of ten people between the ages of 80 and 89 years

B. Terminology. A number of terms are used in association with atrial fibrillation.
1. **"Valvular"** refers to atrial fibrillation that is due to valve disease, most commonly **rheumatic mitral valve disease.** In the past, rheumatic heart disease accounted for most cases of atrial fibrillation, but currently it accounts for less than one-third of cases.
2. **"Isolated"** refers to atrial fibrillation that is secondary to another illness (e.g., hyperthyroidism, pneumonia, pulmonary embolism) and resolves when the illness is treated.
3. **"Paroxysmal"** refers to intermittent episodes of atrial fibrillation unrelated to an acute illness.
4. **"Chronic"** refers to atrial fibrillation when it is the predominant rhythm for longer than 1 month.
5. **"Lone"** refers to atrial fibrillation in the absence of structural heart disease [e.g., hypertensive heart disease, congestive heart failure (CHF), coronary artery disease (CAD)]. Lone atrial fibrillation accounts for 2%–4% of cases.

II CAUSES OF ATRIAL FIBRILLATION.
Because many causes of atrial fibrillation are correctable, an effort should be made to identify the cause of the arrhythmia.

A. Cardiovascular disorders
1. **Myocardial disorders,** including CAD, hypertensive heart disease, CHF, cardiomyopathy (dilated and hypertrophic), infiltrative heart disease (amyloidosis, sarcoidosis, and hemochromatosis), and myocarditis
2. **Valvular disorders,** including mitral stenosis and endocarditis
3. **Pericardial disorders,** including pericarditis
4. **Congenital heart disease,** including atrial and ventricular septal defects

B. Pulmonary disorders, including pulmonary embolism

C. Metabolic disturbances, including hyperthyroidism and electrolyte disturbances

D. Intoxication (e.g., alcohol, cocaine, theophylline, and β agonists)

E. Infection, including sepsis

F. Stress-induced (e.g., post-surgery)

G. Idiopathic. In less than 5% of patients, no cause can be found; these patients are said to have "lone" atrial fibrillation.

III CLINICAL MANIFESTATIONS OF ATRIAL FIBRILLATION

A. Symptoms are due to loss of the atrial kick and an increased ventricular rate, which results in decreased ventricular filling, decreased cardiac output (CO), and increased myocardial oxygen demand. The most common symptoms reflect these processes.

1. **Dyspnea**
2. **Palpitations**
3. **Lightheadedness or syncope**
4. **Chest pain**
5. **Fatigue**

B. Physical examination findings

1. An **irregularly irregular pulse** is the hallmark of atrial fibrillation.

2. **Pulses vary in intensity** because diastolic filling varies in length and often is reduced. In addition, all audible ventricular beats may not be palpable peripherally.

3. *a* **Waves are absent** in the jugular venous pulse.

4. **The first heart sound (S_1)** varies in intensity.

HOT KEY

Patients with atrial fibrillation never have a fourth heart sound (S_4).

C. Electrocardiography

1. **P waves are absent.**

2. The **ventricular response** will be **irregularly irregular,** although this may be difficult to appreciate at higher heart rates.

3. The electrocardiogram (ECG) may show **f waves** (fine fibrillation of the atria at a rate of 350–600 beats/min), which are visualized best in lead V_1.

IV **APPROACH TO THE PATIENT.** Knowledge of the differential diagnosis will help direct diagnostic testing. All patients should have an ECG, a chest radiograph, a complete blood count (CBC), electrolyte studies, and thyroid function testing. An echocardiogram is usually obtained to examine cardiac function and to rule out valve disease.

V **COMPLICATIONS.** The risk of **stroke** in all patients with atrial fibrillation is approximately 5% per year, 5–7 times the risk in those without atrial fibrillation.

A. **Risk factors for stroke**
   1. **Rheumatic valve disease**
   2. **Older than 60 years**
   3. **Prior stroke**
   4. **CHF**
   5. **Hypertension**
   6. **Left atrial size greater than 5 cm**
B. **Risk assessment for stroke**
   1. In patients with no risk factors, the risk of stroke is approximately the same as the risk in the general population.
   2. If the patient has one or two risk factors, the risk of stroke is approximately 5% per year without anticoagulation therapy.
   3. If the patient has three or more risk factors, the risk increases to roughly 20% per year without anticoagulation therapy.

VI **TREATMENT**

A. **Acute treatment.** The goal of acute treatment of a patient with atrial fibrillation is **rate control.**
   1. **Electrical cardioversion.** Cardioversion is indicated in patients with **rapid atrial fibrillation** who are **unstable** (e.g., with ischemia, severe hypotension, or severe pulmonary edema). Begin immediate cardioversion starting with 100 J in the synchronized mode.
      a. Unless there is an emergent indication, no patient with atrial fibrillation documented longer than 48 hours duration should be cardioverted or receive antiarrhythmic agents. It is safest to first anticoagulate these patients for 4 weeks before cardioversion or to rule out left atrial thrombus with a transesophageal echocardiogram to minimize the risk of stroke.
      b. In patients with electrocardiographically documented atrial fibrillation of less than 48 hours duration, cardioversion can be performed safely without anticoagulation therapy or a transesophageal echocardiogram.

> **HOT**
> **▶**
> **KEY**
>
> The patient's history is often unreliable in determining the on-set of atrial fibrillation. Patients admitted with "new onset" atrial fibrillation should generally be anticoagulated for 4 weeks before electrical or chemical cardioversion.

   2. Pharmacologic therapy
      a. Intravenous atrioventricular (AV) nodal blocking agents (Table 8-1) can slow the ventricular response in patients with rapid atrial fibrillation.
         (1) Digoxin is a good first-line agent.
         (2) β Blockers and **calcium channel blockers** have a much faster onset of action and are useful to rapidly slow the ventricular rate.
         (3) All of these agents should be avoided in patients with irregular, wide-complex tachycardia until atrial fibrillation with conduction down an accessory pathway (e.g., **Wolff-Parkinson-White syndrome**) has been excluded. If Wolff-Parkinson-White syndrome is present with antidromic conduction, these agents can increase the ventricular rate and precipitate ventricular fibrillation.
      b. Intravenous antiarrhythmic agents (Table 8-2) are often necessary in the acute setting to expedite the restoration of normal sinus rhythm. Some agents can also be used to slow the ventricular rate.
         (1) Continuous ECG monitoring is required for patients receiving intravenous antiarrhythmic medication, generally in a coronary care unit (CCU).
         (2) A daily 12-lead ECG should be performed to monitor for QRS and QT prolongation.
   B. Chronic treatment. The goals of chronic treatment of atrial fibrillation are minimization of symptoms and reduction of the risk for stroke.
      1. Rate control. The goal is a resting heart rate lower than 90 beats/min. Treatment should be selected after considering the patient's other medical problems.
         a. In patients with CAD or hypertension, a **β blocker** is appropriate because it treats these disorders as well as the atrial fibrillation. In patients with asthma or severe chronic obstructive pulmonary disease (COPD), however, a **calcium channel blocker,** such as diltiazem or verapamil, may be a better choice to avoid β-blocker-induced bronchoconstriction.
         b. In patients with CHF, **digoxin** can control the heart rate as well as the symptoms of CHF. In patients with chronic renal insufficiency, however, the dose of digoxin should be reduced and the serum digoxin levels monitored closely.

TABLE 8-1. Intravenous Atrioventricular (AV) Nodal Blocking Agents

Drug Class	Dose	Warnings
Digoxin	0.5 mg IV followed by 0.25 mg IV every 6 hours to a total dose of 1 mg	Consider lowering the dose if the patient is elderly, has renal insufficiency, or is taking amiodarone.
β Blockers	Metoprolol: 5 mg IV; dose may be repeated every 5 minutes to a total dose of 15 mg Esmolol: 500 mg/kg IV over 1 minute, followed by an IV maintenance infusion of 50–200 mg/kg/min*	Use with caution in patients with decompensated heart failure; avoid in patients with active bronchospasm.
Calcium channel blockers	Diltiazem: 15–20 mg (0.25 mg/kg) IV over 2 minutes; dose may be repeated in 15 minutes, followed by an IV maintenance infusion of 5–20 mg/hr Verapamil: 2.5–5.0 mg IV over 2 minutes; dose may be repeated with a 5- to 10-mg dose in 15 minutes; maximum dose is 30 mg	Avoid in patients with severe systolic dysfunction

IV = intravenous.
*Because of its short half-life, esmolol can be quickly stopped if hypotension, bradycardia, or bronchospasm occurs.

   c. In patients with inadequate rate control that is refractory to medical therapy, **AV nodal ablation** and **pacemaker implantation** are sometimes used.

  2. Rhythm control. Theoretically, conversion to and maintenance of normal sinus rhythm will reduce the risk of stroke and relieve symptoms related to atrial fibrillation.

   a. Electrical cardioversion should be undertaken after 4 weeks of warfarin anticoagulation with a therapeutic international normalized ratio (INR) of 2.0–3.0. Alterna-

TABLE 8-2. Intravenous Antiarrhythmic Agents

Drug	Dose	Warnings
Procainamide	1 g IV over 1 hour, followed by an IV maintenance infusion of 1–4 mg/min	Consider reducing the dose in patients with renal insufficiency. Monitor for QRS and QT interval prolongation. Also, monitor serum levels of procainamide and its active metabolite NAPA*
Amiodarone	150 mg IV over 10 minutes, followed by an IV maintenance infusion of 1 mg/min for 6 hours, then decreasing to 0.5 mg/min	Consider reducing the dose of digoxin and warfarin.
Ibutilide†	1 mg IV over 10 minutes; dose may be repeated in 15 minutes	Avoid in patients with hypokalemia or a prolonged QT interval, and also in patients on medications that may prolong the QT interval

IV = intravenous; NAPA = N-acetyl procainamide.
*The therapeutic levels are 4–10 mg/mL for procainamide and 15–25 mg/mL for NAPA.
†Ibutilide is most effective in patients with atrial fibrillation of less than 45 days duration, and is a good choice when continued antiarrhythmic therapy is not needed.

tively, a transesophageal echocardiogram can be used to exclude left atrial thrombus, facilitating earlier cardioversion. Warfarin should be continued for another 4 weeks after successful cardioversion.

   b. Pharmacologic therapy can also accomplish cardioversion and is useful for maintaining sinus rhythm after cardioversion. All antiarrhythmic agents, however, have proarrhythmic effects. For each individual patient, the risks of proarrhythmia must be weighed against the risks of stroke from atrial fibrillation.

(1) **Class I_A antiarrhythmics** (see Appendix B for dosing). **Procainamide** and **quinidine** both increase conduction of the AV node (necessitating adequate AV nodal blockade) and are moderately effective in controlling rhythm. Because of the concern for proarrhythmia, these agents should be avoided in patients with structural heart disease (e.g., those with a reduced ejection fraction).

(2) **Class I_C antiarrhythmics. Propafenone** has β blocker effects. As a class I agent, it should be avoided in patients with structural heart disease.

(3) **Class III antiarrhythmics. Amiodarone** and **sotalol,** when compared with class I antiarrhythmics, appear to be more effective in maintaining sinus rhythm. Amiodarone has the lowest risk of proarrhythmia, but has significant side effects (e.g., thyroid dysfunction, pulmonary fibrosis, tremor, corneal deposits) when administered chronically. Baseline thyroid and liver function tests should be performed before the initiation of amiodarone therapy and should be repeated every 6 months.

3. **Clot control.** Stroke is the major cause of morbidity and mortality in patients with chronic atrial fibrillation. Anticoagulation therapy is time-consuming and bothersome to patients, and the risks and benefits must be assessed on an individual basis.

   a. **Warfarin** treatment reduces the risk of stroke by 40%–90%. The target INR should be 2.0–3.0. There is a small increase in the risk of major bleeding (e.g., intracranial and gastrointestinal bleeding). In patients on amiodarone, the dose of warfarin should be decreased by approximately 50%.

   b. **Aspirin** alone is appropriate for patients younger than 60 years with lone atrial fibrillation.

References

Blitzer M, Costeas C, Kassotis J, et al: Rhythm management in atrial fibrillation—with a primary emphasis on pharmacological therapy: Part 1. *Pacing Clin Electrophysiol* 21(3):590–602, 1998.

Golzari H, Cebul RD, Bahler RC: Atrial fibrillation: restoration and maintenance of sinus rhythm and indications for anticoagulation therapy. *Ann Intern Med* 125(4):311–323, 1996.

Jung F, DiMarco JP: Treatment strategies for atrial fibrillation. *Am J Med* 104(3):272–286, 1998.

Mackstaller LL, Alpert JS: Atrial fibrillation: a review of mechanism, etiology, and therapy. *Clin Cardiol* 20(7):640–650, 1997.

Stettin GD: Treatment of nonvalvular atrial fibrillation. *West J Med* 162(4):331–339, 1995.

9. Wide QRS Tachyarrhythmias

....

I **INTRODUCTION.** Ventricular tachycardia and ventricular fibrillation are serious cardiac arrhythmias, which require immediate diagnosis and treatment. Ventricular tachycardia should be distinguished from another cause of wide QRS tachyarrhythmias, such as supraventricular tachycardia with aberrant conduction.

A. Ventricular tachycardia has a wide QRS complex ($\geq$ 0.12 second) and can be categorized by its duration and electrocardiographic pattern.
   1. **Duration**
      a. **A salvo** has 3–5 consecutive beats.
      b. **Nonsustained ventricular tachycardia** has more than 5 beats and continues for less than 30 seconds.
      c. **Sustained ventricular tachycardia** continues for 30 seconds or longer.
   2. **Electrocardiographic pattern**
      a. **Monomorphic ventricular tachycardia** is characterized by a uniform QRS pattern.
      b. **Polymorphic ventricular tachycardia** is characterized by a QRS pattern that changes in its amplitude and axis. The most common form is **torsades de pointes** (i.e., "twisting of the points"), which is characterized by QT prolongation (usually longer than 500 msec) and undulation around the isoelectric point on the ECG.
B. Ventricular fibrillation has an irregularly irregular rhythm and no definite P waves or QRS complexes. The electrocardiogram (ECG) shows chaotic deflections of varying amplitude and contour.
C. Supraventricular tachycardia with aberrant conduction may mimic ventricular tachycardia. Because the treatment of and prognosis for supraventricular tachycardia are different, an accurate diagnosis is important. A 12-lead ECG can usually determine the correct diagnosis.

II **CAUSES OF VENTRICULAR TACHYCARDIA**

A. Causes of monomorphic ventricular tachycardia are listed in order of decreasing frequency:
   1. **Coronary artery disease** (CAD) [e.g., myocardial ischemia and infarction]

2. **Cardiomyopathy** (e.g., dilated, hypertrophic)
3. **Hypertensive heart disease**
4. **Valvular heart disease** (e.g., aortic stenosis, mitral valve prolapse)
5. **Electrolyte imbalance** (e.g., hypokalemia, hyperkalemia, hypomagnesemia) or a **hypercatecholamine state** (e.g., pheochromocytoma)
6. **Drug-induced** (e.g., digoxin toxicity, antiarrhythmics, tricyclic antidepressants, ethanol, cocaine)
7. **Myocarditis**
8. **Infiltrative heart disease** (e.g., amyloidosis)
9. **Trauma** (e.g., myocardial contusion)
10. **Other** (e.g., **right ventricle dysplasia, tetralogy of Fallot**)

B. **Causes of polymorphic ventricular tachycardia**
   1. Polymorphic ventricular tachycardia is caused predominantly by CAD.
   2. The known predisposing factors for **torsades de pointes** are listed in order of decreasing frequency:
      a. **Drug-induced, with quinidine as the most common cause.** Other drugs include class I_A, I_C, and III antiarrhythmics, tricyclic antidepressants, phenothiazines (particularly thioridazine), and pentamidine.
      b. **Electrolyte imbalance** (e.g., hypokalemia, hypomagnesemia, hypocalcemia)
      c. **Central nervous system (CNS) disease** (e.g., subarachnoid hemorrhage)
      d. **Congenital QT prolongation syndrome**

III WIDE, REGULAR TACHYARRHYTHMIAS

A. **Mechanism**
   1. **Normal conduction.** Normally, the impulse is conducted from the sinoatrial (SA) node to the atrioventricular (AV) node, through the bundle of His, through the left and right bundle branches, and through the Purkinje fibers to the myocytes. The bundles conduct rapidly and ventricular depolarization is efficient, producing a narrow QRS complex (< 100 msec in duration).
   2. **Wide QRS complex.** There are two different mechanisms of producing a wide QRS complex:
      a. The QRS complex will be wide if the **impulse starts in the ventricle** and spreads muscle fiber to muscle fiber (as is the case with ventricular tachycardia).
      b. The QRS complex will be wide if **the impulse starts above the ventricle but eventually spreads fiber to fiber** (as is the case with supraventricular tachycardia with aberrancy). There are three mechanisms of aberrant conduction:

    (1) A preexisting bundle branch block. If one bundle is blocked, conduction will spread down the remaining bundle and then from fiber to fiber. This slow process produces a wide QRS complex (> 120 msec). A QRS complex between 100 and 120 msec in duration may represent an incomplete bundle branch block and often is termed an interventricular conduction delay (IVCD).

    (2) A rate-related bundle branch block. As the heart rate increases, one bundle (usually the right bundle) is unable to keep up with the other. The impulse is conducted down the faster bundle and then from fiber to fiber, producing a wide QRS complex.

    (3) An accessory pathway. These tracts terminate in ventricular muscle, necessitating fiber-to-fiber conduction (e.g., Wolff-Parkinson-White syndrome).

B. Differential diagnosis. The **Brugada criteria** can help you distinguish between ventricular tachycardia and supraventricular tachycardia with aberrancy (Table 9-1). Examine the precordial leads (V_1–V_6) on a 12-lead ECG. If a criterion is met, ventricular tachycardia is diagnosed. If the criterion is not met, continue to the next criterion.

    1. Absence of a true RS pattern in all of the precordial leads. If there is a monomorphic pattern with no **RS complex,** the arrhythmia is ventricular tachycardia.

    2. RS complex (from start of R to nadir of S) is greater than 100 msec. Ventricular depolarization takes more time if it starts in the ventricle, rather than if it begins supraventricularly and is conducted aberrantly. If the RS complex is greater than 100 msec, then the arrhythmia is ventricular tachycardia.

    3. Evidence of AV dissociation includes P waves marching through at a different rate than the QRS complex rate.

TABLE 9-1. Classification of Wide QRS Tachyarrhythmias

Regular Rhythm	Irregular Rhythm
Ventricular tachycardia	Atrial fibrillation with aberrancy*
Supraventricular tachycardia with aberrancy	Ventricular tachycardia (monomorphic† or polymorphic)

*Atrial flutter with variable block and multifocal atrial tachycardia with aberrancy must also be considered here, although they are much less common than atrial fibrillation.

†The first 50 beats of monomorphic ventricular tachycardia may be irregular.

Fusion or capture beats also suggest ventricular tachycardia. If a diagnosis still has not been reached, morphologic criteria can be used to arrive at a diagnosis.

HOT KEY Patients with known cardiac disease presenting with a wide QRS tachyarrhythmia should be assumed to have ventricular tachycardia until proven otherwise.

C. Treatment. It is important to rule out easily reversible causes (e.g., an electrolyte abnormality, hypoxemia) of ventricular arrhythmias first. A careful review of current medications is also very helpful.

HOT KEY Sodium bicarbonate (1 mEq/kg intravenously) may be useful if the ventricular tachycardia is a result of hyperkalemia, acidosis, or a tricyclic antidepressant overdose.

1. **Hemodynamically unstable (or ischemic) patients** should undergo immediate **electrical cardioversion** starting at 200 J.
2. **Hemodynamically stable patients**
   a. **Ventricular tachycardia**
      (1) **Acute therapy**
         (a) **Lidocaine.** The initial dose is 1–1.5 mg/kg administered as a bolus intravenously. This dose can be repeated in 5 minutes followed by a continuous infusion of 1–4 mg/min.
         (b) **Procainamide** should be considered in patients who do not respond to lidocaine. The initial dose is 17 mg/kg administered intravenously over 1 hour followed by a continuous infusion of 2–4 mg/min.
         (c) **Amiodarone** should be considered if the patient remains in ventricular tachycardia. The initial dose is 150 mg administered intravenously over 10 minutes, followed by 1 mg/min for 6 hours, then 0.5 mg/min.
      (2) **For long-term treatment** of life-threatening ventricular tachycardia or ventricular fibrillation, consider class III antiarrhythmic therapy (e.g., amiodarone, sotalol) and possibly an automatic implantable cardiac defibrillator for high-risk patients.
   b. **Supraventricular tachycardia with aberrancy. Carotid sinus massage** and **adenosine** should be employed as described in Chapter 7 II B 1 b.

IV WIDE, IRREGULAR TACHYARRHYTHMIAS

A. Differential diagnosis. The main differential diagnosis is **ventricular tachycardia** (monomorphic or polymorphic) versus **atrial fibrillation with aberrancy** (see Table 9-1).
1. **Ventricular tachycardia**
   a. **Monomorphic ventricular tachycardia.** The rhythm may be irregular for the first 50 beats. A persistently irregular rhythm after 50 beats essentially rules out monomorphic ventricular tachycardia.
   b. **Polymorphic ventricular tachycardia.** Because the impulse is originating from different foci in the ventricle, the rhythm is irregular.
2. **Atrial fibrillation with aberrancy.** There are three possible mechanisms of aberrant conduction:
   a. **A preexisting bundle branch block.** If there is evidence of an old bundle branch block on a previous 12-lead ECG that has the same morphology as the present one, this diagnosis is extremely likely.
   b. **A rate-related bundle branch block** will usually have a right bundle branch block pattern on the ECG because the right bundle conducts slower than the left bundle.
   c. **An accessory pathway.** If there is evidence of preexcitation during sinus rhythm (i.e., a short PR interval with delta waves) on a prior 12-lead ECG, this diagnosis is extremely likely. Atrial fibrillation accompanied by an accessory pathway is a dangerous situation because atrial fibrillatory waves occur at rates of approximately 600 beats/min and the accessory pathway allows much faster conduction than does the AV node. Very fast ventricular rates (i.e., 200–300 beats/min) can occur; this arrhythmia can quickly degenerate to ventricular fibrillation.

 HOT KEY Whenever you see a patient with a wide, irregular tachyarrhythmia with a rate greater than 200 beats/min, consider atrial fibrillation with conduction down an accessory pathway.

B. Treatment
1. **Hemodynamically unstable (or ischemic) patients** should undergo immediate **electrical cardioversion** starting at 200 J.
2. **Hemodynamically stable patients**
   a. **Monomorphic ventricular tachycardia** is treated as described in III C 2 a.

b. Polymorphic ventricular tachycardia

    (1) Stop offending drugs (e.g., class I_A antiarrhythmics, tricyclic antidepressants, phenothiazines) and **correct electrolyte abnormalities.**

    (2) Consider administering magnesium sulfate (2 g intravenously over 1 minute), even if the serum magnesium level is normal.

    (3) Consider increasing the heart rate to 100–120 beats/min with **isoproterenol** or **overdrive cardiac pacing** to terminate torsades de pointes.

c. Atrial fibrillation with aberrancy

    (1) If preexisting or rate-related bundle branch block causes the aberrancy, then treatment should be instituted as described in Chapter 8 VI A.

    (2) If there is evidence of an accessory pathway, **do not administer AV nodal blocking agents (e.g., β blockers, calcium channel blockers, digoxin).** These AV nodal blockers may promote conduction down the accessory tract, thereby increasing the ventricular rate. The drug of choice is **procainamide,** which will slow conduction through the pathway and decrease the ventricular rate.

References

Antiarrhythmics Versus Implantable Defibrillators (AVID) Investigators. A comparison of antiarrhythmic-drug therapy with implantable defibrillators in patients resuscitated from near-fatal ventricular arrhythmias. *N Engl J Med* 337(22): 1576–1583, 1997.

Brugada P, Brugada J, Mont L, et al: A new approach to the differential diagnosis of a regular tachycardia with a wide QRS complex. *Circulation* 83(5):1649–1659, 1991.

Delbridge TR, Yealy DM: Wide complex tachycardia. *Emerg Med Clin North Am* 13(4):903–924, 1995.

Hamdan M, Scheinman M: Current approaches in patients with ventricular tachyarrhythmias. *Med Clin North Am* 79(5):1097–1120, 1995.

Shah CP, Thakur RK, Xie B, et al: Clinical approach to wide QRS complex tachycardias. *Emerg Med Clin North Am* 16(2):331–360, 1998.

10. Cardiac Pacemaker Therapy

I **INTRODUCTION.** Approximately one million people in the United States have a permanent pacemaker. Primary care physicians frequently evaluate patients who have or may require a permanent pacemaker. Therefore, it is important to understand how pacemakers function, the options for pacemaker programming, and the indications and complications associated with permanent pacing.

II **TYPES OF PACING**

A. Transcutaneous pacing may be performed in unstable patients who need emergent pacing until a transvenous pacemaker can be inserted. The pacing pads are applied to the patient's chest, and the pacemaker is programmed. Because this procedure is usually uncomfortable, intravenous analgesics and sedatives are often used.

B. Temporary transvenous pacing is used in unstable patients who require immediate pacemaker therapy (e.g., those with bradycardia or pause-dependent torsades de pointes). A fluoroscope is often used to advance the pacing lead through the internal jugular, subclavian, or femoral vein and into the right ventricular apex.

C. Permanent pacing involves the surgical implantation of a device into the patient's body and is used for patients who require chronic pacemaker therapy. Typically, the patient receives local anesthesia so that the pulse generator (see III B) can be placed in a "pocket" overlying the pectoralis major muscle in the subclavian region. The leads are then inserted into the subclavian vein and advanced into the heart using a fluoroscope.

    1. Dual-chamber pacemakers generally require two separate leads: one to the right atrium and one to the right ventricle.

    2. A new single-lead system involves one lead that allows ventricular sensing and pacing in addition to atrial sensing.

III **PERMANENT PACEMAKER COMPONENTS.** The modern permanent pacemaker is a complex instrument. Failure of any of the following components may result in pacemaker malfunction:

A. The lithium battery, which lasts 5–15 years depending on how often the pacemaker initiates a paced beat

B. The pulse generator, which includes the circuits and a micro-computer chip that dictates how the pacemaker will operate

C. The sealed housing, which is a small container (approximately 5 to 7 mm thick) that encloses the battery and pulse generator and keeps the circuitry dry

D. The lead system, which consists of insulated wires that connect the sealed housing to the electrodes (which have tined or "screw-in" tips attached to the endocardial surface of the heart during implantation)

IV **PACEMAKER PROGRAMMING.** In the United States, roughly two- thirds of the pacemakers used are dual cham-ber, two-thirds are rate adaptive, and one-third have both ca-pabilities. Modern pacemakers have a number of **program-mable features,** including the pacing mode, rate, output, sensitivity, and rate adaptation.

A. The **pacing mode** is the most important feature for the primary care physician.

  1. The **pacing code** is composed of three to five letters (Table 10-1).

   a. The first letter denotes the chamber that is paced.

   b. The second letter denotes the chamber that is sensed.

   c. The third letter indicates the type of response [e.g., inhib-ited (I), activated or triggered (T), or both (D)] that the pacemaker makes to a sensed signal.

   d. The fourth letter indicates other programmable features, such as rate modulation.

   e. The fifth letter indicates the pacemaker's antitachycardia pacing and shocking capabilities. It is generally reserved for automatic implantable cardioverter defibrillators (AICDs).

  2. Choosing a pacing mode. Although many different pacing modes exist (Table 10-2), the following two modes are en-countered most frequently.

   a. The **DDD mode** is the most versatile pacing mode.

    (1) Methodology. The DDD mode senses and paces both the atrium and ventricle; therefore, during exercise, the ventricular rate will increase if the sinus rate in-creases. If atrial arrhythmias exist, the pacemaker can be programmed not to "track" any arrhythmias above a maximum ventricular rate, thereby preventing a rapid ventricular rate from occurring in response to atrial fibrillation or flutter.

    (2) Indications. The DDD mode is useful for patients

TABLE 10-1. Pacing Code Positions

I	II	III	IV	V
Chambers paced	**Chambers sensed**	**Response to sensing**	**Programmable functions**	**Antitachyarrhythmia functions**
A = atrium	A = atrium	T = triggers	P = programmable*	P = pacing†
V = ventricle	V = ventricle	I = inhibits	M = multiprogrammable‡	S = shock
D = dual (A + V)	D = dual (A + V)	D = dual (T + I)	C = communicating (telemetry)	D = dual (P + S)
O = none	O = none	O = none	R = rate adaptation	O = none
			O = none	

*Programmable rate, output, or both.
†Programmable rate and output for antitachycardia pacing.
‡Multiprogrammable rate, output, and sensitivity.

TABLE 10-2. Commonly Used Pacing Modes

I Chambers paced	II Chambers sensed	III Response to sensing	IV Programmable functions	Description
D	D	D	...	Paces and senses in atrium and ventricle; paces the ventricle in response to sensed atrial activity up to the programmed upper rate limit
D	D	D	R	Same as DDD, plus change in atrial and ventricular rates in response to sensor output
V	V	I	...	Demand ventricular pacing; output inhibited by sensed ventricular signals
V	V	I	R	Same as VVI, plus ventricular rates can change in response to sensor output
A	A	I	...	Demand atrial pacing; output inhibited by sensed atrial signals

A = atrium; D = dual; I = inhibits; R = rate responsive; V = ventricle.

with sinus node dysfunction and atrioventricular (AV) node disease.

b. VVI mode

(1) Methodology. The VVI mode paces and senses the ventricle only, providing "ventricular pacing on demand."

(2) Indications. The VVI mode is most useful for patients who have chronic atrial fibrillation and severe AV node disease, and need ventricular pacing only.

B. The **rate** can be programmed to detect the lower rate limit, which is the minimal intrinsic heart rate tolerated before pacing begins. Dual-chamber pacemakers can also be programmed for the upper rate limit, which is the maximal heart rate at which the atrial rate is tracked in a 1:1 relationship.

C. The **output** determines the amount of energy generated by the pacemaker when it delivers a paced beat.

D. The **sensitivity** refers to the amplitude of the intracardiac signal that will be sensed as intrinsic atrial or ventricular activity.

E. The **rate adaptation** feature allows the pacing rate to be increased during exercise. Sensors are designed so that the pulse generator can mimic the response of the normal heart rate when the metabolic need is increased during exercise. Typically, these sensors can detect motion (using a piezoelectric crystal) or minute ventilation (by tracking the changes in thoracic impedence).

HOT

KEY

When a magnet is placed over the pulse generator, the mode for single-chambered ventricular pacemakers switches to VOO and the mode for dual-chamber pacemakers switches to DOO (pacing without sensing). Changing to a pacing without sensing mode is useful when a patient's pacemaker is inappropriately sensing stimuli leading to pacemaker inhibition.

V **INDICATIONS FOR PERMANENT PACING.** In addition to specific electrocardiographic criteria for permanent pacemaker therapy, medical and psychosocial factors (e.g., the patient's overall health and preference, concerns expressed by family members) should be considered when evaluating a patient for permanent pacemaker therapy. Pacemaker therapy may be appropriate for patients with the following disorders:

A. Sinus node dysfunction (i.e., sick sinus syndrome) broadly refers to sinus bradycardia, sinus arrest, and paroxysmal tachycardia (i.e., tachycardia–bradycardia syndrome). Patients who report symptoms (e.g., lightheadedness, syncope) during episodes of significant bradycardia (i.e., heart rate slower than 45 beats/min) may be considered for pacemaker implantation.

B. AV block

1. Patients with third-degree (complete) AV block are generally considered candidates for pacemaker therapy.

2. Patients with second-degree Mobitz type II AV block or symptomatic Mobitz type I block (i.e., Wenckebach block) may also be considered for pacing.

C. Fascicular block. Impaired conduction in the left or right bundles below the AV node may progress to complete heart block, necessitating permanent pacing. The conduction system is composed of three fascicles: the right bundle, the left anterior fascicle (see Chapter 2 IV C 1 a), and the left posterior fascicle (see Chapter 2 IV C 2 e). If there is abnormal conduction in two or three of these fascicles, **bi- or trifascicular block** (respectively) is present. Pacemaker therapy may be considered for patients with bi- or trifascicular block who have symptoms (e.g., syncope).

D. Carotid sinus hypersensitivity. Patients with recurrent syncope and a diagnosis of carotid sinus hypersensitivity (where carotid sinus massage results in asystole that lasts longer than 3 seconds) may be considered for pacemaker therapy.

E. Cardiomyopathy. Pacemaker therapy for patients with cardiomyopathy is under investigation.

1. **Dilated cardiomyopathy.** In patients with dilated cardiomyopathy that is refractory to medical therapy, trials are currently being performed to determine whether dual-chamber pacing with a short AV interval may improve the patient's symptoms and increase cardiac output (CO).

2. **Hypertrophic cardiomyopathy.** In patients with severe hypertrophic cardiomyopathy that is refractory to medical therapy, there is already evidence that dual-chamber pacing with a short AV interval can decrease the left ventricular outflow tract gradient and improve symptoms.

F. Acute myocardial infarction (AMI). In patients with AMI, guidelines for permanent pacing remain controversial.

1. **Anterior wall infarction.** In patients with a new bifascicular block, second-degree AV block and bundle branch block, or third-degree AV block, a pacemaker is generally indicated because extensive conduction disease is likely.

2. **Inferior wall infarction.** Because the prognosis for patients with inferior wall infarction is not adversely affected by AV block or bundle branch block, patients with transient high grade AV block are generally not considered for permanent pacing.

VI **COMPLICATIONS** associated with pacemaker therapy include:

A. Hemorrhage, venous thrombosis, pericardial effusion and tamponade, pneumothorax, and infection following pacemaker implantation
B. Erratic pacing or sensing, which can be caused by pacing electrode migration

---

HOT

Magnetic resonance imaging (MRI) is generally contraindicated in pacemaker patients.
KEY

VII **FOLLOW-UP** includes assessment of the battery status, pacing threshold, sensing function, and lead integrity.

A. **Transtelephonic testing.** Pacemaker surveillance programs can assess pacemaker function over the telephone.
B. **Clinic appointments** are generally scheduled 2 weeks following pacemaker implantation (for a wound check) and then annually. Patients who are dependent on a pacemaker typically have follow-up evaluations scheduled every 3–6 months. More frequent visits should be scheduled close to the end of the pacemaker battery's life.

References

Gregoratos G, Cheitlin MD, Conill A, et al: ACC/AHA Guidelines for Implantation of Cardiac Pacemakers and Antiarrhythmia Devices: Executive Summary—report of the American College of Cardiology/American Heart Association Task Force on Practice Guidelines (Committee on Pacemaker Implantation). *J Am Coll Cardiol* 31(5):1175–1206, 1998.

Hayes DL, Barold SS, Camm AJ, et al: Evolving indications for permanent cardiac pacing: an appraisal of the 1998 American College of Cardiology/American Heart Association Guidelines. *Am J Cardiol* 82(9):1082–1086, 1998.

Kusumoto FM, Goldschlager N: Cardiac pacing. *N Engl J Med* 334(2):89–97, 1996.

Mitrani RD, Myerburg RJ, Castellanos A: Cardiac pacemakers. In *Hurst's The Heart,* 9th ed. Edited by Alexander RW, Schlant RC, Fuster V, et al. New York, McGraw-Hill, 1998, pp 1023–1055.

PART III

CORONARY ARTERY DISEASE

11. Chest Pain

I **INTRODUCTION.** Because chest pain (including "discomfort") is common and its etiologies range from life-threatening myocardial infarction (MI) to benign musculoskeletal pain, a simple and reliable approach to the patient is necessary.

II **CAUSES OF CHEST PAIN.** One way to remember the causes of chest pain is to use an "outside–in" approach.

A. Skin. Varicella-zoster virus infection (shingles) often causes pain before vesicular lesions are noted. The pain usually occurs in a dermatomal distribution.

B. Chest wall. Musculoskeletal pain may result from shoulder arthritis or bursitis, intercostal injury, metastatic bone or chest wall disease, or costochondritis. Breast pathology (e.g., tumors, fibrocystic disease) and nerve root compression (from cervical disk herniation) may also lead to chest pain.

C. Lungs. Inflamed pleura from pneumothoraces, pulmonary emboli, infections, malignancies, and connective tissue disorders can all cause chest pain, which is usually pleuritic (i.e., it worsens with inspiration or coughing).

D. Heart and great vessels. Pericarditis, myocardial ischemia and infarction, and aortic dissection can all cause chest pain.

E. Gastrointestinal tract. Esophageal disorders (including esophagitis, spasm, and rupture), gastric and duodenal ulcers, pancreatitis, and biliary disease are common causes of chest pain.

III **APPROACH TO THE PATIENT.** Although the outside-in approach is useful in remembering the differential diagnoses for chest pain, it fails to highlight the four acutely life-threatening causes:

HOT

KEY

4 Killer Chest Pains
MI
Aortic dissection
Pulmonary embolism
Spontaneous pneumothorax

Because chest pain may represent one of these emergencies, the usual order of evaluation (e.g., history, physical examination, diagnostic tests) may hinder critical early intervention. The first step should be a quick screen for the four killer chest pains, followed by a more in-depth evaluation if the etiology remains unclear.

A. **Screen for the killer chest pains.**
   1. **"Eyeball" the patient.** A patient who is clutching the chest and appears diaphoretic and ashen can be diagnosed presumptively with acute myocardial infarction (AMI) from across the room. Even if the presentation is not so classic, you can often decide on who "looks sick," and may need a more rapid evaluation in a more monitored setting.
   2. **Establish intravenous access and cardiac rhythm monitoring** immediately in patients who appear ill or who have cardiac risk factors.

HOT

KEY

Any abnormality of the vital signs should alert you to the possibility that the chest pain has a potentially serious cause.

---

   3. **Evaluate the patient's vital signs.**
      a. **Check the blood pressure in both arms.** Although a difference in systolic blood pressure of 10 mm Hg or more may be seen in patients with aortic dissection, local atherosclerosis can also produce pressure differences. Therefore, the blood pressure reading does not rule in or rule out aortic dissection.
      b. **Check the respiratory rate and oxygen saturation.** Low oxygen saturation may accompany pneumothorax, pulmonary embolism, pneumonia, and MI (with pulmonary edema).
         (1) A **low oxygen saturation** (e.g., $\leq 92\%$) is often an indication that oxygen therapy should be started, and an arterial blood gas should be ordered.
         (2) A **normal oxygen saturation** may still be accompanied by a significant alveolar-atrial (A-a) oxygen gradient

during hyperventilation. Therefore, arterial blood gas testing may still be necessary to evaluate the possibility of pulmonary embolism if the rest of the evaluation is unrevealing.

4. **Look at the electrocardiogram (ECG).**
   a. **ECG abnormalities** that suggest **MI** or **ischemia** should signal an admission. (The emergent management of AMI is discussed in Chapter 12.) If the ECG findings indicate new right axis deviation (RAD), right ventricular hypertrophy (RVH), right atrial enlargement, or right bundle branch block (RBBB), **pulmonary embolism** should be suspected.
   b. **Normal ECG.** Because a normal ECG does not rule out MI or ischemia, **nitroglycerin** (0.4 mg sublingually or via aerosol) may be administered and the dose repeated every 3–5 minutes as both a diagnostic challenge and as potential therapy.

HOT KEY

In patients with a history of coronary artery disease (CAD) or cardiac risk factors and no alternative explanation for the chest pain after careful evaluation, an admission to rule out myocardial infarction (ROMI) is usually appropriate.

---

5. **Take a preliminary history.**
   a. **Cardiac history and risk factors.** First, ask about any prior cardiovascular problems.
      (1) If there is a history of CAD, the patient has ischemia until proven otherwise.
      (2) With a negative cardiac history, you can quickly establish the initial probability of MI by assessing cardiac risk factors (i.e., age, male sex, smoking, diabetes, hypertension, hypercholesterolemia, and positive family history).
   b. **Other risk factors.** The preliminary history can also identify any other predisposing factors to the killer chest pains. For example, a history of cancer or inactivity may lead to pulmonary embolism, and uncontrolled hypertension may increase the likelihood of aortic dissection or MI.
6. **Perform a preliminary physical examination.** Frequently, you will have a few brief moments between tests where you can look at the neck veins, listen to the lungs and heart, palpate the abdomen for tenderness, and evaluate the pulses and warmth in the extremities.
7. **Evaluate the chest radiographs.** Always compare the new films to old films, if they are available.
   a. Spontaneous pneumothorax can be subtle and you need to look carefully, especially in the apices.

      b. Esophageal rupture may lead to air in the mediastinum (pneumomediastinum).

      c. MI or aortic dissection may be accompanied by enlargement of the heart or mediastinum, respectively. The presence of pulmonary edema may also be suggestive of AMI.

B. Further define the cause of the chest pain.

  1. Take a more detailed history.

      a. Type of chest pain. Pulmonary embolism frequently presents with pleuritic chest pain. MI may present with "crushing" substernal chest pain or only a mild "discomfort." Aortic dissection is often characterized by a "ripping" pain of severe intensity.

      b. Radiation of chest pain. Pain that radiates to the neck, jaw, or left arm should be considered cardiac until proven otherwise. Pain that radiates to the back often is associated with aortic dissection.

      c. Onset of chest pain. Spontaneous pneumothorax, pulmonary embolism, and aortic dissection usually present with abrupt pain, whereas pain from MI or ischemia may build more gradually. Spontaneous pneumothorax and pulmonary embolism often occur while the patient is at rest, whereas aortic dissection and MI may occur with rest or exertion.

      d. Duration of chest pain. Pain that only lasts seconds or that has been constant for more than 24 hours is usually not caused by one of the four killer chest pains. An AMI is almost always associated with more than 20 minutes of chest pain.

      e. Associated symptoms. Dyspnea, diaphoresis, lightheadedness, or syncope should alert you to a probable serious cause of chest pain.

      f. Aggravating and mitigating factors

        (1) Deep inspiration often aggravates pain from the pleura or pericardium (e.g., pleurisy from a pulmonary embolism or pericarditis).

        (2) Exertion may worsen the pain from MI or aortic dissection. Rest may ease the pain from cardiac ischemia, usually gradually.

        (3) Position. Patients with pericarditis often feel worse when supine and better sitting up. Patients with musculoskeletal pain and esophageal reflux may feel worse in certain positions (e.g., supine or bending over to tie shoes). Position usually does not affect the pain of MI.

        (4) Food intake. Pain on swallowing localizes the problem to the gastrointestinal tract. Chest pain after a meal may indicate gastrointestinal pathology, but it may also occur with MI.

(5) Nitroglycerin. If chest pain decreases with nitrates (e.g., sublingual nitroglycerin), a cardiac etiology should be presumed; however, esophageal spasm may also respond to this therapy.

2. Perform a complete physical examination.

   a. Jugular venous pressure. An elevated jugular venous pressure should alert you to the possibility of a serious disorder (e.g., MI, pulmonary embolism, or tension pneumothorax), but a normal jugular venous pressure does not exclude these disorders.

   b. Cardiac examination (see Chapter 1)

      (1) Heart sounds. Listen carefully for a third heart sound (S_3) or fourth heart sound (S_4), which may indicate impaired ventricular contractility or relaxation, respectively. Both abnormal ventricular contractility and abnormal relaxation can accompany myocardial ischemia.

      (2) Murmurs may also increase the likelihood of a cardiac etiology of chest pain. A mitral regurgitant murmur may accompany MI with papillary muscle ischemia. An aortic insufficiency murmur may accompany an ascending aortic dissection. An ejection murmur may indicate aortic stenosis or hypertrophic cardiomyopathy (both conditions predisposing the patient to ischemia).

   c. Lung examination. Listen carefully for rales (e.g., from MI with pulmonary edema) and pleural friction rubs (e.g., from pulmonary embolism, infection, or other pleural processes).

   d. Chest wall examination. Minimal tenderness to palpation is nonspecific, but if the chest pain is exactly and reliably reproduced, a musculoskeletal etiology is likely.

   e. Abdominal examination. Palpate for abdominal tenderness that may indicate a gastrointestinal cause of the chest pain.

   f. Pulses. Check the pulses in the arms and legs bilaterally.

3. Pearls

   a. MI

      (1) Because CAD is common and potentially life-threatening, it is always better to admit patients for ROMI if any doubt exists as to the diagnosis, even in young patients.

      (2) More than 20 minutes of unexplained chest pain may represent AMI, whereas chest pain that lasts less than 20 minutes but increases in frequency, duration, or occurs with minimal exertion often represents unstable angina; both patterns are indications for admission.

      (3) Frequently, patients with chest pain are given an antacid and lidocaine swish and swallow ("GI cocktail") to evaluate possible reflux esophagitis. Keep in mind, however, that patients who "benefit" from this "diagnostic test" may actually have ischemic pain that is improving spontaneously or from bed rest and oxygen therapy.

b. Aortic dissection

   (1) The greater curvature of the aorta is the site for most dissections; therefore, the right coronary artery is involved most frequently. If the patient has a sudden onset of severe pain radiating to the back, unequal blood pressures, or other suspicious findings (e.g., hypertension or aortic insufficiency) accompanied by evidence of acute inferior MI, aortic dissection should be considered.

   (2) Transesophageal echocardiography (TEE), computed tomography (CT), and magnetic resonance imaging (MRI) are used in the evaluation of aortic dissection (Figure 11-1). The choice of diagnostic

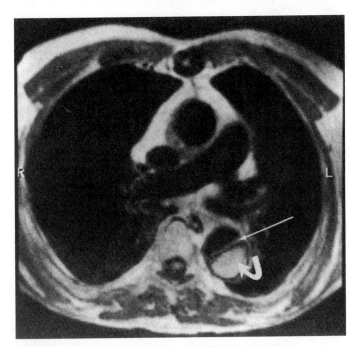

FIGURE 11-1. Aortic dissection diagnosed by magnetic resonance imaging (MRI). The intimal tear (*straight arrow*) and the contrast-filled false lumen (*curved arrow*) can be seen. (Courtesy of C. Higgins, M.D., San Francisco, CA)

modality depends chiefly on institutional preferences and which test can be completed most efficiently. If clinical suspicion is high, a surgeon should be consulted immediately.

c. Pulmonary embolism. Clinical suspicion is critical because there is often no clinical evidence of deep vein thrombosis. If clinical suspicion is high, administer heparin intravenously before sending the patient for diagnostic tests (e.g., ventilation-perfusion scan or pulmonary angiography).

d. Spontaneous pneumothorax. An end-expiratory chest radiograph may demonstrate a subtle pneumothorax.

References

Jesse RL, Kontos MC: Evaluation of chest pain in the emergency department. *Curr Probl Cardiol* 22(4):149–236, 1997.

O'Rourke RA: Chest pain. In *Hurst's The Heart,* 8th ed. Edited by Alexander RW, Schlant RC. New York, McGraw-Hill, 1994, pp 459–468.

Zalenski RJ, Shamsa F, Pede KJ: Evaluation and risk stratification of patients with chest pain in the emergency department: Predictors of life-threatening events. *Emerg Med Clin North Am* 16(3):495–517, 1998.

12. Angina Pectoris

I INTRODUCTION

A. Definition. Angina is the symptom of **chest pain** that results when the oxygen supply is inadequate to meet the oxygen demands of the cardiac muscle. Although other diseases may reduce the oxygen supply (e.g., coronary artery spasm, hypoxia, anemia) or increase the oxygen demand (e.g., tachycardia as a result of infection, thyrotoxicosis), angina rarely occurs without **underlying coronary artery disease (CAD).**

B. Risk factors for CAD include:
1. Age greater than 45 years for men or 55 years for women
2. Male sex
3. Diabetes mellitus
4. Smoking habit
5. Hypercholesterolemia
6. Hypertension
7. Family history (i.e., CAD in a first-degree male relative younger than 55 years or a female relative younger than 65 years)

C. Classification. Angina may be **stable** or **unstable.**
1. **Stable angina** usually results from a fixed atherosclerotic plaque that limits oxygen delivery to the myocardium. When oxygen demand increases (e.g., from physical exertion or emotional stress), the oxygen supply cannot be increased to compensate. The resulting oxygen mismatch causes a predictable and stable pattern of chest pain during exertion.
2. **Unstable angina** usually occurs when an atherosclerotic plaque ruptures and becomes thrombosed. As a result, the oxygen supply is inadequate at lower activity levels, and sometimes even at rest.

II CLINICAL MANIFESTATIONS OF CAD

A. Symptoms
1. **Angina** is usually experienced beneath or left of the midsternum, increases with physical exertion or stress, often lasts from a few minutes up to 20 minutes, and subsides gradually with rest or nitroglycerin.
   a. The quality of angina is often described as squeezing, burning, or as a dull pressure sensation.
   b. If chest pain radiates to the neck or left arm or is accompanied by dyspnea, diaphoresis, or lightheadedness, the

likelihood that the pain represents angina is increased. These features, however, need not be present.

   c. Symptoms of stable angina occur predictably, whereas symptoms of unstable angina increase in frequency or duration or occur with less exertion (even at rest).

  2. **"Anginal equivalents."** Other symptoms unaccompanied by chest pain (e.g., dyspnea) actually may represent "anginal equivalents." Some patients with CAD may not have any symptoms at all.

B. Signs on physical examination

  1. Because patients often have no discernible signs of illness, a normal physical examination does not rule out the possibility of CAD.

  2. Transient signs may occur during ischemic episodes and include:

    a. Hypertension or, less commonly, hypotension

    b. Ventricular arrhythmias

    c. A third or fourth heart sound (S_3 or S_4)

    d. A holosystolic murmur over the apex (representative of mitral regurgitation as a result of papillary muscle ischemia)

  3. The presence of elevated jugular venous pressure, pulmonary edema, or signs of cardiac risk factors (e.g., peripheral vascular disease from diabetes) should all increase suspicion of CAD.

III APPROACH TO THE PATIENT. Stable and unstable angina must be differentiated from the many other causes of chest pain (see Chapter 11).

A. Patient history. In patients with classic symptoms, the diagnosis of stable or unstable angina can be made on the basis of history alone.

B. Resting electrocardiogram (ECG). Unstable angina also can be diagnosed by finding evidence of active ischemia on a resting ECG (e.g., ST-segment depressions or T-wave inversions).

C. Stress tests may be helpful both diagnostically in patients with atypical chest pain and prognostically in patients with typical stable angina (see Chapter 4). Stress testing is usually contraindicated in patients with suspected unstable angina.

  1. Types

    a. Exercise electrocardiography. The presence of 1 mm of down-sloping or horizontal ST-segment depression, or 2 mm of up-sloping ST-segment depression is considered a positive test for exercise-induced myocardial ischemia.

    b. Myocardial perfusion scintigraphy is often performed in conjunction with exercise electrocardiography and involves the intravenous administration of thallium-201 or technetium-99m sestamibi. Cardiac muscle cells that are ischemic or infarcted do not take up the nuclear isotopes normally.

    (1) Additional information is generated by comparing the scintigraphic images obtained directly after exercise and at rest.

        (a) Reversible defects, areas that lack isotope on exercise images but "fill in" on resting images, indicate ischemia.

        (b) Fixed defects do not change on resting images and usually denote myocardial infarction (MI).

    (2) In patients who are unable to exercise, vasodilators, such as **dipyridamole** or **adenosine,** are used. These agents produce greater vasodilation in normal coronary arteries than in atherosclerotic vessels, thereby causing the isotope to shunt away from cardiac regions served by diseased vessels. Dipyridamole and adenosine are contraindicated in patients with active bronchospasm.

  c. Stress radionuclide angiography or echocardiography. If exercise or pharmacologic stress decreases the left ventricular ejection fraction (LVEF) or results in segmental wall motion abnormalities, cardiac ischemia is presumed. Intravenous **dobutamine** increases oxygen demand by increasing heart rate and contractility and may be used as an alternative to exercise in stress echocardiographic studies.

2. Choosing a test. Although one stress test cannot be universally recommended over the others, two caveats apply:

  a. Patients with baseline ECG abnormalities [e.g., left bundle branch block (LBBB), left ventricular hypertrophy (LVH) with repolarization abnormality, digoxin effect] may not be evaluated appropriately with standard exercise electrocardiography alone.

  b. Echocardiography is usually not an adequate test in obese patients because of suboptimal imaging.

D. Coronary angiography is necessary to definitively diagnose CAD (see Chapter 5).

1. Stable angina. Because stable angina can usually be diagnosed on the basis of the patient history or noninvasive studies, coronary angiography usually is not needed for diagnosis; rather, it is usually performed to help determine subsequent therapy. In patients with markedly abnormal stress tests or who remain symptomatic after appropriate medical therapy, coronary angiography is performed to determine whether revascularization with coronary artery bypass graft surgery (CABG) or percutaneous coronary intervention (PCI) is needed (see IV B 2).

2. Unstable angina. Coronary angiography is indicated in patients with unstable angina who have complications while in the hospital [e.g., recurrent angina or congestive heart failure (CHF)] or an abnormal stress test.

IV TREATMENT

A. **General measures.** Because angina indicates underlying CAD, an essential part of the treatment plan is aimed at identifying and treating cardiac risk factors.
   1. **Smoking cessation**
   2. **Weight loss**
   3. **Regular exercise** (e.g., brisk walking for 30 minutes 4 times weekly)
   4. **Control of hypercholesterolemia** [low-density lipoproteins (LDL) goal < 100 mg/dl]. HMG-CoA reductase inhibitors are generally considered the drugs of choice.
   5. **Control of hypertension** (systolic blood pressure < 140 mm Hg, diastolic blood pressure < 90 mm Hg)
   6. **Control of diabetes**
   7. **Treatment of other factors that may aggravate angina** (e.g., anemia, hypoxia, thyrotoxicosis)

B. **Specific measures for the relief of stable angina**
   1. **Pharmacologic therapy** is generally aimed at increasing the myocardial oxygen supply (by coronary vasodilation) and decreasing the oxygen demand (by decreasing heart rate, contractility, preload, or afterload). Most patients are started on aspirin, a β blocker, and nitrates unless there are contraindications.
      a. **Aspirin** (usually 325 mg/day) inhibits platelet aggregation and coronary thrombosis, and may therefore decrease the risk of unstable angina and MI.
      b. **β Blockers** reduce heart rate and contractility, resulting in symptomatic control of angina. In addition to preventing cardiac arrhythmias, these agents also have a mortality benefit in patients who have already experienced MI.
         (1) In general, the dose of the β blocker may be increased until symptoms are controlled, side effects develop (e.g., postural lightheadedness), blood pressure falls below approximately 100/60 mm Hg, heart rate falls below approximately 50 beats/min, or the maximal dose is reached.
         (2) Frequently used β blockers include **propranolol, metoprolol,** and **atenolol** (see Appendix B for dosing).
         (3) **β blockers are contraindicated** in patients with bradyarrhythmias, conduction disease, or overt CHF.
            (a) In patients with chronic obstructive pulmonary disease (COPD), a β_1-selective agent (e.g., metopro-

lol or atenolol) should be used; often, all β blockers are avoided in patients with severe COPD.

(b) Patients with impaired left ventricular systolic function may actually benefit the most from β blockers; however, candidates must have well-compensated heart failure (i.e., no evidence of pulmonary edema or jugular venous distention) before therapy is initiated. The patient should be started with a low dose (e.g., 3.125 mg of metoprolol or carvedilol two times daily), which is gradually increased with frequent patient monitoring.

c. Nitrates increase oxygen supply by vasodilating the coronary arteries, and decrease oxygen demand by decreasing preload and afterload.

(1) Short-acting nitrates. Nitroglycerin (0.3–0.6 mg sublingually or by aerosol) may be used for **immediate therapy** or **angina prophylaxis**.

(a) Immediate therapy. The dose is administered every 3–5 minutes until the pain is relieved; if the pain is not relieved in 15 minutes, the patient should get to the nearest hospital immediately.

(b) Angina prophylaxis. The dose is taken 5 minutes before an activity known to result in angina.

(2) Long-acting nitrates (e.g., isosorbide dinitrate, isosorbide mononitrate, transdermal nitroglycerin patches). A nitrate-free interval of approximately 8–10 hours per day is needed to prevent tachyphylaxis. Headaches frequently occur with the initiation of nitrate therapy; they can be managed conservatively and frequently resolve within 1–2 weeks.

d. Calcium channel blockers lower oxygen demand (by decreasing heart rate, contractility, and afterload) and may increase oxygen supply (by inducing vasodilation of the coronary arteries). Although calcium channel blockers are not the initial drugs of choice for most patients with angina, they are used in symptomatic patients who are not improving with β blockers and nitrates.

(1) Agents include **nifedipine, diltiazem,** and **verapamil,** in order of decreased effect on lowering systemic vascular resistance and increased effect on myocardial inotropy and chronotropy.

(2) Calcium channel blockers have not been associated with improved survival post-MI, and may lead to a worse outcome.

(3) Newer calcium channel blockers, such as amlodipine, felodipine, and isradipine may be safer choices for patients with stable angina.

HOT

KEY

Short-acting nifedipine should be avoided when treating patients with angina.

    2. **Revascularization.** Methods include **PCI** and **CABG.** Coronary angiography should be performed only in patients who are candidates for one of these procedures.
        a. The **indications** for revascularization are controversial. Candidates include:
            (1) Patients with stable angina refractory to medical therapy
            (2) Patients with unstable angina or MI who have recurrent angina, CHF, or an abnormal stress test
        b. **CABG** is generally considered the treatment of choice for patients with left main CAD (stenosis > 50%) or three-vessel disease (stenosis > 70%) associated with depressed left ventricular systolic function (ejection fraction < 50%). CABG is preferred in diabetic patients with multivessel coronary disease because the risk of restenosis and renal complications is lower than that associated with PCI.
C. Specific measures for relief of unstable angina. Patients with unstable angina require admission and should undergo serial cardiac enzyme studies, 12-lead ECGs, and continuous telemetry to rule out acute MI. Patients with active chest pain or ECG evidence of ischemia are always managed in the coronary care unit (CCU). Patients with resolved chest pain and no ECG evidence of ischemia are often treated and monitored in a telemetry unit.
    1. **Pharmacologic therapy** is aimed at inhibiting progression of the presumed intracoronary thrombus and improving the myocardial oxygen mismatch.
        a. **Aspirin** (usually 325 mg/day) is almost always used in patients with unstable angina.
        b. **Heparin** should be used in patients with suspected myocardial ischemia, unless there are contraindications. Unfractionated heparin may be administered intravenously, whereas **low-molecular-weight heparin** (e.g., enoxaparin) may be administered subcutaneously.
        c. **Nitrates** are generally given transdermally or intravenously so that the dose can be titrated carefully to prevent ischemia and to control blood pressure.
            (1) Transdermal nitrates are often used for patients in telemetry units. Table 12-1 outlines a sliding scale for dosing that could be used.
            (2) **Intravenous nitroglycerin** is often used for patients in the CCU. The initial dose is 10 μg/min, which may be

TABLE 12-1. Sliding Scale for Dosing of Nitropaste*

Systolic Blood Pressure (mm Hg)	Dosage
< 100	Wipe off nitropaste
100–120	1 inch every 4 hours
121–140	2 inches every 4 hours
> 140	3 inches every 4 hours

*Appropriate dosing may vary based on the target blood pressure goal and the patient's response to therapy.

titrated up to 200 µg/min to keep the patient symptom-free and the systolic blood pressure at approximately 100–120 mm Hg.

    (3) Long-acting nitrates may be substituted after the patient has stabilized (often after 24–48 hours).

  d. β Blockers should be administered to patients without contraindications, and are especially useful in patients with tachycardia or hypertension.

    (1) Although oral therapy is often sufficient, **intravenous administration of metoprolol** (5 mg every 5 minutes, for a total of 3 doses or 15 mg) may provide faster therapy for patients with active ischemia.

    (2) Patients with hemodynamic instability and those with a higher risk of adverse effects from β blockers (e.g., a history of bronchospasm or depressed left ventricular function) may benefit from an **esmolol intravenous drip** that allows rapid dose titration or discontinuation of therapy.

  e. Glycoprotein IIb/IIIa inhibitors are a new class of antiplatelet agents currently under investigation in the treatment of unstable angina. In high-risk patients, intravenous short-acting agents (e.g., tirofiban or eptifibatide) may be helpful.

HOT KEY

Calcium channel blockers are of unproved benefit and may be deleterious in the management of unstable angina.

  2. Revascularization

    a. Urgent coronary angiography and revascularization should be performed in patients with ongoing chest pain despite maximal medical therapy.

    b. Coronary angiography and revascularization should also be performed in patients who have recurrent angina.

    c. In patients who have an uncomplicated hospital course, a predischarge stress test should be performed; only those patients who show evidence of inducible ischemia should be referred for coronary angiography.

References

Schlant RC, Alexander RW: Diagnosis and management of patients with chronic ischemic heart disease. In *Hurst's The Heart,* 9th ed. Edited by Alexander RW, Schlant RC, Fuster V. New York, McGraw-Hill, 1998, pp 1275–1306.

Théroux P, Waters D: Diagnosis and management of patients with unstable angina. In *Hurst's The Heart,* 9th ed. Edited by Alexander RW, Schlant RC, Fuster V. New York, McGraw-Hill, 1998, pp 1307–1344.

13. Acute Myocardial Infarction

I **INTRODUCTION.** Acute myocardial infarction (AMI) is a leading cause of death in the United States. The failure to recognize AMI in the emergency room has led to inappropriate patient discharges and significant delay in treatment, resulting in an abundance of malpractice claims. Many therapies have a definite mortality benefit in the management of AMI; however, numerous studies show that patients frequently receive suboptimal therapy.

II **PATHOPHYSIOLOGY OF AMI**

A. **Common causes.** AMI usually results from **coronary artery disease (CAD)**. The rupture or thrombosis of atherosclerotic coronary plaques leads to inadequate blood flow and oxygen delivery, which in turn leads to myocardial ischemia and eventually cell death (Figures 13-1 and 13-2).

B. **Rarer causes** of AMI include:
   1. Vasospasm (usually associated with CAD)
   2. Thromboemboli (from mitral valve disease, or left ventricular or left atrial thrombi)
   3. Aortic dissection (usually with right coronary artery involvement)
   4. Vasculitis
   5. Cocaine use (as a result of vasospasm, increased platelet aggregation, or both)
   6. Severe hypotension, anemia, or hypoxemia

III **CLINICAL MANIFESTATIONS OF AMI.** Typical symptoms and signs associated with myocardial ischemia are discussed in Chapter 11 III B. The **chest pain** associated with AMI differs from that of stable angina in that it may begin while at rest, lasts more than 20 minutes, is more severe, and is unrelieved with nitroglycerin. Chest discomfort lasting longer than 20 minutes should be considered due to AMI until proved otherwise. Occasionally, patients with AMI do not present with chest pain, and instead report nausea, jaw or shoulder pain, or shortness of breath.

IV **DIAGNOSIS.** Because AMI and unstable angina share similar pathophysiology, they sometimes are difficult to distin-

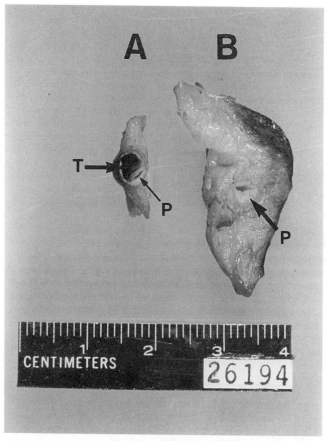

FIGURE 13-1. Cross-sections of the epicardial coronary arteries show atherosclerosis in a patient who has died of acute myocardial infarction (AMI). Both autopsy specimens (A and B) were taken from the same patient. In specimen A, an atherosclerotic plaque (P) ruptured, resulting in thrombosis (T), coronary occlusion, and AMI. In specimen B, a severe atherosclerotic plaque (P) caused significant lumen narrowing; however, it had not ruptured. (Courtesy of P.C. Ursell, M.D., San Francisco, CA)

guish based on clinical criteria alone. Patients are often admitted for "unstable angina/rule out myocardial infarction (ROMI)." Serial electrocardiograms (ECGs) and cardiac enzyme studies are required for a definitive diagnosis. Occasionally, other testing procedures, such as echocardiography,

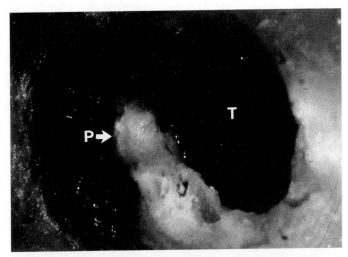

FIGURE 13-2. Magnified cross-section of a coronary artery showing a ruptured atherosclerotic plaque (*P*) and extensive coronary thrombosis (*T*). Inadequate blood flow and oxygen delivery resulted in fatal myocardial infarction (MI). (Courtesy of M.J. Davies, M.D., London UK)

nuclear scintigraphy, and angiography, are also performed to confirm the diagnosis.

> **HOT**
> ▶
> **KEY**
>
> The diagnosis of AMI is made when at least two of the following criteria are present:
> Typical signs and symptoms
> ECG changes
> Elevated cardiac enzymes

A. **Typical signs and symptoms.** Chest pain is the most common symptom of AMI, but other signs and symptoms may also signal AMI (e.g., pulmonary edema, hypotension, nausea, dyspnea).

B. **ECG changes.** AMI is usually associated with **ST-segment elevations** (reflecting transmural myocardial injury) and **pathologic Q waves** (reflecting myocardial necrosis) [see Chapter 2 VII B, VIII B; and Figure 13-3].

C. **Elevated cardiac enzymes**
   1. AMI is usually associated with an elevation in serum creatine kinase (CK) levels. Detection of the CK-MB isoenzyme

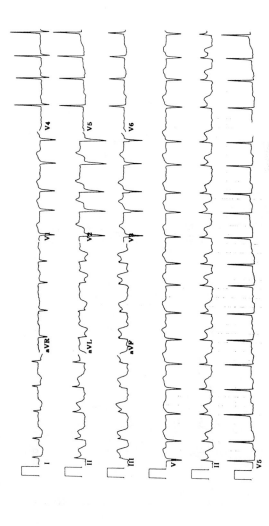

FIGURE 13-3. A 12-lead electrocardiogram (ECG) of a 45-year-old man admitted to the hospital with an acute inferior and right ventricular myocardial infarction (MI). **(A)** Note the ST-segment elevation in the inferior leads (II, III, and aVF). A large inferior MI usually results in reciprocal ST-segment depression in the precordial leads (see V_2). Lead V_1 overlies the right ventricle. The right ventricular MI causes ST-segment elevation in Lead V_1 which averages with the reciprocal ST-segment depression in the anterior precordial leads, resulting in an isoelectric ST segment in lead V_1. *(continued)*

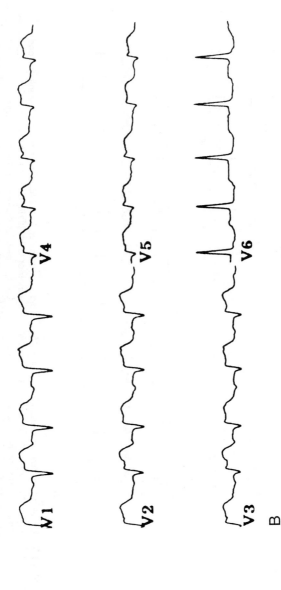

FIGURE 13-3. (*B*) Right-sided leads V$_{4-5}$ show significant ST-segment elevation and confirm the presence of a right ventricular infarction. (Courtesy of G. Thomas Evans Jr., M.D., University of California San Francisco, San Francisco, CA)

has increased specificity for cardiac muscle and maintains a high sensitivity. Studies that measure CK-MB levels are usually ordered every 8 hours for 24 hours or until a peak level is reached.

2. More recently, **troponin levels** have been introduced as a more sensitive and specific means of diagnosing AMI. Troponin levels are checked every 12 hours for 24 hours or until a peak level is reached.

V **APPROACH TO THE PATIENT.** The acute management of patients with AMI requires both precision and speed. The following stepwise approach will allow you to make critical treatment decisions immediately, followed by those that are less urgent. Whenever a patient is evaluated with AMI, it is helpful to answer three questions: What is the patient's hemodynamic status? Is immediate reperfusion therapy [i.e., with thrombolysis or percutaneous coronary intervention (PCI)] indicated? What other treatments may benefit the patient?

A. **What is the patient's hemodynamic status?**
   1. **Assessment.** Hemodynamic status can be approximated by checking the blood pressure and examining the lungs and extremities.
      a. **Low-risk patients** have a normal systolic blood pressure (i.e., > 100 mm Hg). These patients also have clear lungs without rales, indicating normal left ventricular filling pressures [i.e., normal pulmonary capillary wedge pressure (PCWP)]. Warm extremities and normal peripheral pulses imply adequate cardiac output (CO).
      b. **Intermediate-risk patients** have a normal systolic blood pressure and normal extremity examination. On pulmonary examination, however, rales are found in less than 50% of the lung fields, and an elevated left ventricular filling pressure (i.e., a PCWP > 18 mm Hg) is suspected.
      c. **High-risk patients** are in **cardiogenic shock.** These patients often are hypotensive, have rales in at least 50% of the lung fields, and cool extremities with diminished arterial pulses. The presence of pulmonary edema suggests that the PCWP is elevated. Because the CO is low, the patient's blood pressure is low and end organs are inadequately perfused.
   2. **Management**
      a. **Low-risk patients** are hemodynamically stable and have a low mortality rate. Management of these patients entails deciding if immediate reperfusion therapy is indicated, and what other forms of therapy might benefit the patient (see V B, C).

b. Intermediate-risk patients have evidence of pulmonary edema, which may decrease oxygenation while increasing oxygen demand (increased sympathetic tone increases the heart rate and myocardial contractility).

    (1) Intravenous furosemide should be given as needed.

    (2) Nitrates and morphine may also be given to treat pulmonary edema by decreasing preload.

c. High-risk patients

    (1) Pulmonary artery (PA) line placement is indicated for monitoring CO, systemic vascular resistance, and PCWP.

    (2) Pharmacologic therapy is dictated by the patient's systemic blood pressure. Although **hypotension** often accompanies cardiogenic shock, the blood pressure may still be normal with low flow states due to a marked increase in systemic vascular resistance.

HOT

KEY

Do not assume that a normal blood pressure indicates adequate end-organ perfusion.

    (a) Systolic blood pressure lower than 100 mm Hg. Intravenous **dopamine** is usually the first drug administered to patients in cardiogenic shock. Dopamine often causes **renal artery dilatation** at doses of 1–2 μg/kg/min ("renal dose" dopamine), **increased contractility** from β_1-receptor stimulation at doses of 5–10 μg/kg/min, and **vasoconstriction** from α_1-receptor stimulation at doses of 10–20 μg/kg/min; however, significant overlap and variation exists. Once the systolic blood pressure is higher than 100 mm Hg, dobutamine is often added. Because tachyarrhythmias may complicate dopamine and dobutamine therapy, patients require careful rhythm and electrolyte monitoring (especially of the potassium and magnesium levels).

    (b) Systolic blood pressure higher than 100 mm Hg

      (i) Dobutamine is usually started intravenously at a dose of 2.5 μg/kg/min. The dose may be increased gradually (up to a maximum of 20 μg/kg/min) until the CO rises and the PCWP falls to less than 18 mm Hg. Dobutamine raises the CO by increasing contractility and by decreasing the systemic vascular resistance. Higher doses of dobutamine may cause excessive tachycardia, thus limiting the escalation of the dose.

HOT KEY

A decrease in blood pressure may occur with dobutamine therapy, so the systolic blood pressure usually should be higher than 100 mm Hg before the initiation of therapy.

    (ii) Sodium nitroprusside can effectively reduce systemic vascular resistance. Because nitroprusside causes a decrease in blood pressure, a higher starting blood pressure is often required.
  (3) Emergent PCI is the only therapy that has been shown to decrease mortality in patients in cardiogenic shock.
  (4) Intra-aortic balloon pump (IABP) insertion may also be useful in patients with severe pump failure, persistently poor coronary flow, or both.

B. Is reperfusion therapy indicated? Patients with chest pain of 6 hours or less duration (and possibly up to 12 hours or longer) and ST elevations of at least 1 mm in two consecutive ECG leads [or evidence of new left bundle branch block (LBBB)] should undergo primary PCI or thrombolysis unless there are contraindications.

1. Primary PCI is favored in centers that can perform the procedure quickly and with expertise, and when there are contraindications to thrombolytic therapy. Patients who have **cardiogenic shock, prior coronary artery bypass grafting,** or **recent angioplasty** do not benefit as much from thrombolysis, and should therefore undergo primary PCI.

2. Thrombolysis
  a. Contraindications
    (1) Absolute contraindications generally include:
      (a) Central nervous system (CNS) disease. Recent trauma or surgery, aneurysms, arteriovenous malformations, tumors, or a history of hemorrhagic stroke at any time or nonhemorrhagic stroke within 3 months are usually considered contraindications.
      (b) Active gastrointestinal or **genitourinary bleeding**
      (c) Pregnancy or active menstruation
    (2) Relative contraindications generally include:
      (a) Traumatic or **prolonged cardiopulmonary resuscitation**

    (b) Recent trauma or **surgery** (within 2 weeks)
    (c) Diabetic retinopathy
    (d) Sustained hypertension (e.g., blood pressure $>$ 180/120 mm Hg)
    (e) Coagulopathy, thrombocytopenia, or **current oral anticoagulation therapy**
    (f) Noncompressible arterial or **venous puncture sites**

b. Agents. The two most commonly used thrombolytic agents are **streptokinase** and **tissue plasminogen activator (t-PA).**

  (1) t-PA. Front-loaded t-PA has been found to have a 1% 30-day mortality benefit compared with streptokinase.

    (a) Front-load the dose of t-PA by administering 15 mg/kg in an intravenous bolus, then 0.75 mg/kg (up to 50 mg/kg) over 30 minutes, then 0.5 mg/kg (up to 35 mg/kg) over the next 60 minutes. Because t-PA has a short half-life, intravenous heparin must also be given during or following therapy to decrease the reocclusion rate.

    (b) Advantages. t-PA is preferred for patients who have had a recent streptococcal infection or received streptokinase within the last 6 months. Because t-PA causes less hypotension than streptokinase, it may also be preferred for patients with borderline blood pressure. t-PA may provide additional benefits to certain patient subgroups, such as young patients with anterior wall MI who present within 4 hours of the onset of symptoms.

  (2) Streptokinase

    (a) The usual **dose** is 1.5 million units administered intravenously over 1 hour.

    (b) Advantages. Streptokinase has a slightly lower incidence of hemorrhagic stroke than t-PA (0.5% versus 0.7%–0.8%). Elderly patients and those with elevated blood pressure (i.e., a systolic blood pressure $>$ 160 mm Hg) have a higher risk of hemorrhagic stroke; therefore, streptokinase may be the preferred agent in these patients. In addition, streptokinase is less expensive than t-PA.

  (3) Newer thrombolytic agents include reteplase and tenecteplase (TNK). These agents are similar to t-PA in structure, and may eventually replace t-PA because they are easier to administer and may be more effective and safer for the patient.

  c. **Signs of successful reperfusion** include a prompt decrease in the severity of chest pain, at least a 50% improvement in the degree of ST- segment elevation, an accelerated idioventricular rhythm, and an early peak of the CK enzymes (within 12 hours). If these clinical criteria are not met within 90 minutes, **rescue PCI** should be considered.

C. **What other treatments may benefit the patient?** Specific forms of therapy with nitrates and β blockers are outlined in Chapter 12. The **coronary care unit (CCU)** is the best place to manage patients with AMI, given the need for frequent vital checks, continuous rhythm monitoring, intravenous medications, and prompt defibrillation for life-threatening ventricular arrhythmias.

  1. **General measures**
     a. **Bed rest** and a **stool softener** are usually prescribed.
     b. **Subcutaneous heparin** (5000 units twice daily) is administered to prevent deep venous thrombosis, unless the patient is already receiving intravenous standard heparin or subcutaneous low-molecular-weight heparin.
     c. **Analgesia. Nitrates** and **morphine sulfate** (4–8 mg intravenously) are usually given to relieve pain.
     d. **Oxygen** (2–4 L/min) is often administered, although the benefit in patients with normal oxygen saturation is questionable.

  2. **Aspirin** (usually 325 mg orally) has been shown to have a mortality benefit, even in patients who receive thrombolytics.

  3. **β blockers** have been shown to decrease mortality in patients with AMI, and are particularly useful in patients with tachycardia or hypertension. Contraindications include hypotension, bradycardia, high-grade atrioventricular (AV) block, and active bronchospasm.

  4. **Angiotensin-converting enzyme (ACE) inhibitors** have been shown to have a mortality benefit in patients with AMI. Administering ACE inhibitors early (i.e, within 24 hours of the onset of symptoms) offers additional benefit. Patients most likely to benefit from ACE inhibitors are high-risk patients with CHF and anterior wall MI. Contraindications include hypotension, hyperkalemia, bilateral renal artery stenosis, and possibly severe renal insufficiency.

  5. **Nitrates** are usually given unless the patient is hypotensive or has evidence of right ventricular MI.

  6. **Intravenous heparin** is useful in patients with AMI who are being treated with t-PA or primary PCI.

> **HOT**
> ▶
> **KEY**
>
> Calcium channel blockers have not been shown to have a mortality benefit in patients with AMI, and in some studies have been associated with increased mortality. Diltiazem may decrease the reinfarction rate in patients with non-Q wave MI, but may not decrease mortality. In general, these agents should be avoided in the management of AMI.

VI COMPLICATIONS

A. Arrhythmias are most common during the initial 12–24 hours after AMI.

  1. Tachyarrhythmias are evaluated and treated as discussed in Chapters 7 and 9.

    a. Prophylactic lidocaine is associated with higher rates of asystole and a poorer outcome and is no longer recommended. Lidocaine is usually used for patients with sustained ventricular tachycardia or fibrillation, and may be considered for patients with frequent or symptomatic episodes of nonsustained ventricular tachycardia.

    b. Prophylactic magnesium is also not recommended; it is reserved for patients with polymorphic ventricular tachycardia.

  2. Bradyarrhythmias are more common with inferior wall AMI because the sinoatrial (SA) and AV nodes are more dependent on blood flow from the right coronary artery.

    a. Atropine (0.5–1 mg administered intravenously every 3–5 minutes, up to 3 mg) is usually effective for severe sinus bradycardia and symptomatic Mobitz type I block.

    b. Temporary pacing is generally indicated for patients with AMI and:

      (1) Symptomatic sinus bradycardia and Mobitz type I block that is unresponsive to atropine

      (2) Mobitz type II block or third-degree AV block

      (3) New bifascicular block, including alternating left and right bundle branch block, RBBB with left anterior fascicular block or posterior fascicular block, and LBBB with first-degree AV block

B. Recurrent ischemia following AMI is usually an indication for **emergent coronary angiography** and **revascularization.**

C. Pump dysfunction. Severe left ventricular failure is managed as outlined for high-risk patients in cardiogenic shock (V A 2 c). An **IABP** or a **left ventricular assist device** may also be considered until more definitive therapy (i.e., cardiac transplantation) can be carried out.

D. Right ventricular infarction should always be suspected when hypotension accompanies an inferior AMI. Treatment involves

large fluid boluses to increase right-sided filling pressures and CO. **Inotropic agents** with hemodynamic monitoring may also be required. Nitrates and diuretics should be avoided.

E. **Mechanical complications** usually occur 2–7 days following AMI.

  1. **Cardiac tamponade** from **rupture of the left ventricular free wall** usually leads to sudden hypotension and death.

  2. **Ventricular septal defect (VSD)** or **papillary muscle rupture leading to acute mitral regurgitation**

     a. The **clinical signs and symptoms** include pulmonary edema, hypotension, or both. Any abrupt change in hemodynamics should increase clinical suspicion of one of these mechanical complications.

     b. The **physical examination** reveals a new holosystolic murmur in both conditions. The murmur location is at the left sternal border in VSD and at the apex in papillary muscle rupture.

     c. **Diagnosis.** An **emergent echocardiogram** can quickly confirm the diagnosis. Hemodynamic monitoring with a PA line is usually necessary for treatment, and may also be used diagnostically. An increased oxygen saturation between the right atrium and pulmonary artery is seen with the left-to-right shunting in VSD. Both disorders may display prominent v waves on the PCWP tracing.

     d. **Treatment.** Nitroprusside or IABP insertion may decrease afterload, thereby increasing the fraction of blood ejected into the aorta compared with the regurgitant fraction ejected into the right ventricle or left atrium. **Emergent surgical repair** is usually indicated for definitive therapy.

  3. **Left ventricular aneurysm** or **pseudoaneurysm**

     a. **Left ventricular aneurysm** most often occurs after large anterior wall MIs. **Warfarin therapy** for 3–6 months is often administered to patients to prevent thromboembolism. Left ventricular aneurysms may be associated with refractory heart failure or ventricular arrhythmias, and may require **surgical correction**.

     b. **Pseudoaneurysms** are distinguished by a relatively narrow neck and a predisposition for an inferior–posterior location. The ventricular wall is composed of only thrombus and pericardium; **surgical correction** is generally performed to prevent delayed rupture.

 RISK STRATIFICATION. The major cardiac complications following AMI include CHF, recurrent ischemia and infarction, and life-threatening ventricular arrhythmias. In order to reduce the risk of these complications, diagnostic testing is aimed at identifying patients at increased risk. Chapter 14 reviews the strategies of secondary prevention in survivors of AMI.

A. **CHF.** The postinfarction left ventricular ejection fraction (LVEF) is an excellent predictor of future complications and survival. For this reason, patients usually receive a test to measure the LVEF (e.g., an echocardiogram, left ventriculogram, or nuclear medicine wall motion study) before discharge from the hospital.

B. **Myocardial ischemia.** Patients with postinfarction angina or ST depression on a resting ECG are at increased risk for reinfarction. These high-risk patients are generally referred for early coronary angiography and revascularization. Stress testing to screen for patients with residual ischemia is recommended for the remaining patients.

1. **Stress testing** (see Chapter 4) is useful for identifying high-risk patients who may need early coronary angiography and revascularization. The addition of imaging modalities (e.g., echocardiography or nuclear imaging techniques) can increase the diagnostic accuracy of stress tests.

   a. **Symptom-limited exercise treadmill testing** can be conducted safely in appropriate patients before hospital discharge.

   b. For patients unable to exercise, **pharmacologic stress testing** (i.e., with dipyridamole, dobutamine, or adenosine) can be performed.

2. **Coronary angiography with revascularization** is usually indicated for patients with abnormal stress tests that show significant myocardial ischemia (particularly in high-risk patients with non-Q wave MI, depressed LVEF, and ventricular arrhythmias).

C. **Ventricular arrhythmias**

1. **Patient risk.** Sudden death accounts for more than 50% of all deaths during the first year in survivors of AMI. A variety of testing strategies are available to identify patients at increased risk for sudden death due to ventricular tachycardia or fibrillation.

HOT

KEY
Ventricular arrhythmias that only occur within 24 hours of AMI generally do not require chronic antiarrhythmic therapy.

---

   a. **Patients with sustained ventricular tachycardia or symptomatic nonsustained ventricular tachycardia** (i.e., three or more consecutive ventricular premature beats lasting less than 30 seconds) more than 24 hours after AMI generally require antiarrhythmic treatment.

b. **High-risk patients** [e.g., those with a reduced LVEF, abnormal signal-averaged ECG (SAECG), or abnormal invasive electrophysiologic study] usually require further testing and additional treatment because they are at an increased risk for sudden death.

c. **Low-risk patients** (e.g., those with a normal LVEF and a normal SAECG) do not necessarily benefit from additional treatment.

2. **Treatment**

a. **Amiodarone** is the only antiarrhythmic medication that is generally considered safe to administer in postinfarction patients. Amiodarone is generally considered for patients who are suspected to be at high-risk for sudden cardiac arrhythmic death. The proarrhythmic effects associated with all other agents may actually increase the risk of sudden death in survivors of AMI.

b. **Automatic implantable cardioverter defibrillators (AICDs)** can be used either alone or in combination with amiodarone to treat recurrent ventricular tachyarrhythmias. Studies have shown that AICDs may offer a superior mortality benefit (as compared with amiodarone) in the treatment of high-risk patients following AMI.

References

Alexander RW, Roberts R, Pratt CM: Diagnosis and management of patients with acute myocardial infarction. In *Hurst's The Heart,* 9th ed. Edited by Alexander RW, Schlant RC, Fuster V. New York, McGraw-Hill, 1998, pp 1345–1434.

The GUSTO Investigators: An international randomized trial comparing four thrombolytic strategies for acute myocardial infarction. *N Engl J Med* 329:673–682; 1993.

Muller DWM, Topol EJ: Reperfusion therapy for acute myocardial infarction. In *Cardiology: Physiology, Pharmacology, Diagnosis.* Edited by Parmley WW, Chatterjee K. New York, Lippincott, 1995, pp 1–28.

14. Primary and Secondary Prevention

I **INTRODUCTION.** Coronary artery disease (CAD) is the leading cause of death in the United States; therefore, prevention and treatment of CAD is important.

II **PRIMARY PREVENTION** refers to physician efforts aimed at patients with no known CAD. There are two goals:

A. **Prevention of CAD risk factors**
   1. **Tobacco use.** Educate the patient and family about the risks of smoking in adolescents.
   2. **Obesity.** Educate the patient and family about the risks of obesity in young children and significant weight gain in adolescents. Also, encourage patients to maintain an active lifestyle and to follow the American Heart Association's step I diet, which is designed to reduce cholesterol (to < 300 mg/day) and fat intake (total fat to ≤ 30% and saturated fat to < 10%).

B. **Detection and modification of established CAD risk factors**
   1. **Tobacco use.** The goal is **complete cessation.** Provide counseling, nicotine replacement therapy, and referrals to formal cessation programs as necessary.
   2. **Insufficient physical activity.** The goal is for patients to engage in 30 minutes or more of moderate activity 3 to 4 times per week. If patients have limited functional capacity or other serious medical problems, recommend a medically supervised exercise program.
   3. **Obesity.** The goal is for patients to maintain a body weight that is less than 110% of the predicted weight for their particular height and sex (i.e., a body mass index of 21–25 kg/m^2).
   4. **Hypertension.** The goal is a blood pressure less than or equal to **140/90 mm Hg.**
      a. **Lifestyle modifications** include controlling body weight, exercising regularly, eliminating sodium from the diet, and reducing alcohol consumption.
      b. **Pharmacologic therapy** should be initiated if the blood pressure remains greater than or equal to 140/90 mm Hg after 3 months of implementing these lifestyle modifica-

tions, or if the initial blood pressure is greater than 160/100 mm Hg.

5. **Hyperlipidemia**

    a. **Measure the cholesterol levels.** Measure the total cholesterol, low-density lipoprotein (LDL), and high-density lipoprotein (HDL) cholesterol levels in adults older than 20 years and children with a family history of hyperlipidemia or premature CAD.

    b. **Exclude secondary causes of hyperlipidemia,** which include hypothyroidism, nephrotic syndrome, biliary obstruction, hepatoma, chronic renal failure, hyperuricemia, Cushing's syndrome, alcohol abuse, and medications such as steroids, thiazides, and β blockers.

    c. **Determine the treatment goals.**

      (1) The **primary treatment goals** depend on the number of risk factors the patient has for CAD (Table 14-1). CAD risk factors are given in Chapter 12 I B.

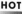

HOT KEY

Primary prevention studies have shown that a 1% reduction in cholesterol reduces the risk of CAD by 2%.

---

      (2) The **secondary treatment goals** are to maintain an HDL level greater than 35 mg/dl and a triglyceride level less than 200 mg/dl.

TABLE 14-1. Guidelines for Treating Hyperlipidemia

Number of CAD Risk Factors*	Primary Treatment Goal LDL Level (mg/dl)	Begin Diet Therapy† LDL Level (mg/dl)	Begin Drug Therapy LDL Level (mg/dl)
0–1	< 160	≥ 160	≥ 190
≥ 2	< 130	≥ 130	≥ 160
Documented CAD	≤ 100	> 100	≥ 130

If the LDL treatment goal is not reached after diet and drug therapies have been initiated, consider combination drug therapy.

CAD = coronary artery disease; LDL = low-density lipoprotein.

*CAD risk factors are listed in Chapter 12 I B.

†American Heart Association's step II diet: ≤ 30% total fat, ≤ 7% saturated fat, < 200 mg cholesterol per day.

TABLE 14-2. Selected Cholesterol-Lowering Medications

Drug	Starting Dose	Maximum Dose	Therapeutic Effects	Indications	Side Effects
Statins* (HMG-CoA reductase inhibitors)			↓ LDL ↑ HDL ↓ TG	First-line drugs for most patients	Elevated liver transaminase, minor increase in CK, myopathy, rhabdomyolysis[†]
Atorvastatin	10 mg daily	80 mg daily			
Pravastatin	10–20 mg daily	40 mg daily			
Lovastatin	20 mg daily	80 mg daily			
Cervistatin	0.2 mg daily	0.4 mg daily			
Simvastatin	20 mg daily	80 mg daily			
Niacin (nicotinic acid)	100 mg twice daily	1–3 g three times daily	↓ VLDL ↓ LDL ↑ HDL ↓ TG	Best drug for increasing HDL levels	Flushing[‡], elevated liver transaminase, worsening of glycemic control (in patients with diabetes), hyperuricemia

	Dosage		Effect	Clinical use	Side effects
Fibric acids			↓ VLDL ↑ HDL ↓ TG	May be useful for patients with very high TG levels	Myalgias, elevated liver transaminase, nausea, abdominal discomfort[§]
Gemfibrozil	300–600 mg twice daily	600 mg twice daily			
Clofibrate	500 mg four times daily	500 mg four times daily			
Resins (bile acid-binders)			↓ LDL	May be useful for patients with elevated LDL levels	Bloating, constipation, vitamin K deficiency[||]
Colestipol	4 g daily	4 g four times daily			
Cholestyramine	2 g daily	4 g four times daily			

CK = creatine kinase; HDL = high-density lipoprotein; HMG-CoA = 3-hydroxy-3-methylglutaryl coenzyme A; LDL = low-density lipoprotein; TG = triglyceride; VLDL = very-low-density lipoprotein.

[*] Statins are most effective when used alone or in combination with niacin or resins.

[†] Check the liver transaminase and CK levels every 4 to 6 months, and stop the medication if the levels rise three times above the upper limit of normal. Avoid administering gemfibrozil or cyclosporine with statins because the combination increases the risk of myopathy.

[‡] Flushing can be prevented by giving the patient aspirin 30 minutes prior to each dose.

[§] If drug interactions occur, decrease the doses of the hypoglycemic and anticoagulant agents.

[||] Drugs in this class impair the absorption of many other medications and should, therefore, be administered 1 hour after these other medications to ensure adequate absorption.

Chapter 14

        d. **Follow the guidelines in Table 14-1** to reach the treatment goal. Drug therapy may be necessary (Table 14-2).
    6. **Diabetes mellitus.** It is not clear whether appropriate glycemic control decreases the risk of CAD development in patients with diabetes. However, aggressive modification of other risk factors (e.g., smoking, hypertension, hyperlipidemia) in patients with diabetes is associated with greater CAD risk reduction than that seen in patients who do not have diabetes but take similar measures.

HOT KEY Aspirin is recommended for patients with a moderate to high risk for CAD, and has been shown to decrease the risk of first myocardial infarction (MI) in men older than 50 years by roughly 40%.

III SECONDARY PREVENTION refers to the treatment methods used in patients with known CAD to reduce the risk of subsequent cardiovascular complications (e.g., MI, stroke, and death).

A. **Lipid control.** In patients with known CAD, more aggressive lipid control is required; the goal is an **LDL level of 100 mg/dl or less**. **Statins** and **niacin** have been shown to decrease the recurrence of MI.

B. **Aspirin** has been shown to decrease mortality and the recurrence of MI, and is recommended for all patients with documented CAD.

C. **β Blockers** reduce the rate of mortality and reinfarction by roughly 25% 1–3 years postinfarction, and by approximately 7% 4–6 years postinfarction.

D. **Angiotensin-converting enzyme (ACE) inhibitors** have been shown to reduce mortality and the recurrence of MI in patients with reduced left ventricular systolic function. They also attenuate ventricular dilatation and remodeling postinfarction.
    1. ACE inhibitors are most effective in patients who have an anterior MI or a left ventricular ejection fraction (LVEF) less than or equal to 40%.
    2. Recent studies have shown that early administration of ACE inhibitors (i.e., within 24 hours of admission) can further reduce mortality in patients who do not have any contraindications (e.g. hypotension, renal artery stenosis, renal insufficiency, hyperkalemia, or angioedema) to this therapy.

E. **Antioxidant vitamins.** Although epidemiologic studies have suggested that beta carotene, vitamin E, and vitamin C may reduce the risk of cardiovascular disease, randomized clinical trials including patients with CAD have not shown a risk reduc-

114

tion. Further studies are necessary to determine the potential cardiovascular benefits and adverse effects of antioxidants.

F. Hormone replacement therapy. Many epidemiologic studies have suggested a benefit of estrogen replacement therapy for postmenopausal women with CAD. Two large, randomized trials, however, investigating estrogen replacement found no significant benefit.

References

Grundy SM, Balady GJ, Criqui MH, et al: Guide to primary prevention of cardiovascular diseases. A statement for healthcare professionals from the task force on risk reduction. American Heart Association Science Advisory and Coordinating Committee. *Circulation* 95(9):2329–2331, 1997.

Michaels AD: The secondary prevention of myocardial infarction. *Curr Prob Cardiol* 24(10):617–680, 1999.

Rackey CE, Schlant RC: Prevention of coronary artery disease. In *Hurst's The Heart*, 8th ed. Edited by Alexander RW, Schlant RC. New York, McGraw-Hill, 1994, pp 1205–1222.

Steering Committee of the Physicians' Health Study Research Group: Final report on the aspirin component of the ongoing Physicians' Health Study. *N Engl J Med* 321(3):129–135, 1989.

PART IV

CONGESTIVE HEART FAILURE

15. Dyspnea

I **INTRODUCTION.** Dyspnea is a common cause of clinic visits, emergency room visits, and hospital admissions. Patients complain of an uncomfortable awareness of breathing, shortness of breath, or a sensation that breathing is difficult.

II **CAUSES.** Cardiac or pulmonary disease cause most cases of dyspnea; however, other causes should also be considered.

A. **Cardiac**
   1. **Myocardial ischemia** or **infarction.** Dyspnea may occur in the absence of chest discomfort and thus may represent an anginal equivalent.
   2. **Congestive heart failure (CHF).** In patients with left ventricular dysfunction, fluid administration may precipitate progressive dyspnea.
   3. **Tachyarrhythmias** cannot be reliably diagnosed on physical examination; a 12-lead electrocardiogram (ECG) or a rhythm strip is required.
   4. **Pericardial tamponade** is rare but should be considered in patients with right-sided heart failure and no evidence of left-sided heart failure.
   5. **Intracardiac shunting** from an atrial or ventricular septal defect can also cause dyspnea.
   6. **Valvular heart disease** from aortic or mitral stenosis or insufficiency may result in dyspnea.
B. **Pulmonary**
   1. **Pneumothorax** is a sudden event that is often accompanied by very acute dyspnea and pleuritic chest pain. This diagnosis should always be considered in patients with asthma and patients on a ventilator.
   2. **Pulmonary embolism** is often difficult to diagnose. Consider this possibility early in the evaluation of most patients with dyspnea because specialized testing is usually required to confirm the diagnosis, and anticoagulation therapy should be initiated as soon as possible.

3. **Bronchospasm** should be suspected in patients with known asthma or chronic obstructive pulmonary disease (COPD). Wheezing is the hallmark physical finding in these disorders; however, other disorders (e.g., CHF) can also cause the patient to wheeze.

4. **Aspiration** should be suspected in patients with swallowing dysfunction or a diminished level of consciousness.

5. **Pneumonia.** Patients will usually have other symptoms of infection, including fever or hypothermia, chills, or a productive cough.

6. **Upper airway obstruction.** An acute onset of symptoms or localized wheezing should prompt consideration of this diagnosis.

7. **Acute respiratory distress syndrome (ARDS).** These patients are usually hospitalized with another diagnosis and have other serious medical problems.

8. **Interstitial lung diseases** (e.g., sarcoidosis and pulmonary fibrosis) usually present in a chronic, progressive course and require extensive diagnostic testing.

9. **Primary pulmonary hypertension** may present with progressive dyspnea.

C. **Metabolic**

1. **Sepsis.** Dyspnea associated with a respiratory alkalosis may be an early finding in a patient with a severe systemic infection.

2. **Metabolic acidosis** can be diagnosed on the basis of an arterial blood gas.

D. **Hematologic. Anemia** can cause dyspnea, and can be missed on history and physical examination.

E. **Gastrointestinal.** Hepatomegaly, ascites, and abdominal masses can cause diaphragmatic elevation, resulting in decreased lung volumes and dyspnea.

F. **Psychiatric. Anxiety** can be the primary cause of dyspnea; however, a diagnosis of a primary anxiety disorder should be considered only after the more serious possibilities have been excluded. In many patients, dyspnea causes anxiety (not vice versa).

III **APPROACH TO THE PATIENT.** Because such a broad range of etiologies is associated with dyspnea [from life-threatening myocardial infarction (MI) to comparatively benign anxiety], a simple and straightforward approach to diagnosing the patient is necessary. The following strategy focuses on patients with acute dyspnea.

A. **Patient history.** There are four key areas of inquiry:

1. Determine the **speed of onset** of the dyspnea.

2. Identify any **associated symptoms** (e.g., chest pain, chills).
3. Find out **what events occurred immediately before the onset** of the dyspnea (e.g., intense activity, change in medication).
4. Assess the patient's **other medical problems.**

B. **Physical examination.** Focus on five key areas:
   1. **Vital signs.** Markedly abnormal vital signs in a patient with dyspnea may signify impending respiratory failure. Obtain an oxygen saturation immediately.

HOT KEY
A normal oxygen saturation does not exclude the possibility of a serious disorder.

   2. **Cardiac.** Perform a complete examination, focusing on the findings of right-sided and left-sided heart failure.
   3. **Pulmonary.** Pay particular attention to the symmetry of breath sounds and the presence of wheezing or rales.
   4. **Extremities.** Examine the patient for edema (unilateral versus bilateral), clubbing, capillary refill time, and cyanosis.
   5. **Mental status**. Evaluate the patient's mental status.
      a. A markedly depressed level of consciousness may necessitate intubation for airway protection.
      b. The finding of altered mental status as a result of the dyspnea suggests a serious disorder.

C. **Initial diagnostic tests.** The following studies are performed routinely when a patient is dyspneic.
   1. **12-Lead ECG**
   2. **Chest radiograph**
   3. **Arterial blood gas**
   4. **Complete blood count (CBC)**
   5. **Electrolytes and renal panel**

HOT KEY
For patients with asthma, a bedside spirometer quickly provides an accurate assessment of the severity of the airflow obstruction

D. **Diagnostic tests to rule out cardiac or pulmonary disease.** In stable outpatients with chronic dyspnea, the following tests can help rule out the two main causes of dyspnea.
   1. **Rule out cardiac disease.** Exercise treadmill testing, echocardiography, and cardiac catheterization can be used to exclude cardiac disease (see Chapters 4 and 5).

2. **Rule out pulmonary disease.**
   a. **Pulmonary function tests (PFTs)** are useful in differentiating obstructive lung disease from restrictive lung disease, assessing the severity of lung disease, and evaluating the patient's response to therapy.
      (1) **Histamine or methacholine** can be used to induce occult asthma.
      (2) Evaluation of the diffusing capacity of the lungs for carbon monoxide **(DLCO)** can be used to assess for pulmonary vascular disease. For example, a low DLCO is present in emphysema and interstitial lung disease.
   b. **High-resolution computed tomography (HRCT)** can be used for the diagnosis of interstitial pulmonary fibrosis (which has a honeycomb pattern of lung parenchyma), interstitial pneumonitis, sarcoidosis, and tumors.
   c. **Ventilation-perfusion (V/Q) lung scanning** can be used to evaluate for chronic thromboembolic disease in high-risk patients.
   d. **Bronchoscopy with biopsy** is helpful in evaluating possible infectious disorders, malignancies, and inflammatory lung disease.
   e. **Open lung biopsy** is occasionally indicated if a tissue diagnosis is required (usually in the workup of restrictive lung disease).

IV TREATMENT

A. **Supplemental oxygen.** All patients with significant dyspnea should be administered supplemental oxygen (particularly when oxygen saturation is $\leq 88\%$). A history of COPD or carbon dioxide retention should not prevent oxygen therapy for hypoxic patients; however, patients at risk for carbon dioxide retention may be given lower amounts of oxygen initially and should be monitored closely.
B. **Diuretics.** Diuretics may be used for any process associated with excess lung water (e.g., pulmonary edema, ARDS, aspiration, pneumonia).
C. **β Agonists.** Wheezing will likely improve somewhat with nebulized β-agonist therapy. These agents, however, should generally be avoided if myocardial ischemia is diagnosed.
D. **Mechanical ventilation.** The need for intubation should be assessed. Indications for mechanical ventilation include:
   1. Refractory hypoxemia ($PaO_2 < 60$ mm Hg despite maximal oxygen therapy)
   2. Ventilatory failure (generally manifested by an increasing $Paco_2$ despite therapy)

3. Inability to protect the airway (often due to a depressed level of consciousness)

4. Impending upper airway obstruction

V FOLLOW-UP AND REFERRAL

A. Follow-up. Patients undergoing evaluation of dyspnea as outpatients should be seen in the clinic frequently (i.e., approximately weekly) until the cause of the dyspnea is diagnosed. During follow-up visits, smoking cessation counseling should be repeated.

B. Referral. When a clear cause cannot be determined, consultation with a **pulmonologist** is often appropriate. Patients with severe COPD, asthma, or interstitial lung disease may also need to see a pulmonologist.

References

Alexander RW: Dyspnea and fatigue. In *Hurst's the Heart,* 8th ed. Edited by Alexander RW, Schlant RC. New York, McGraw- Hill, 1994, pp 469–474.

Manning HL, Schwartzstein RM: Pathophysiology of dyspnea. *N Eng J Med* 333(23):1547–1553, 1995.

Morgan WC, Hodge HL: Diagnostic evaluation of dyspnea. *Am Fam Physician* 57(4):711–716, 1998.

16. Congestive Heart Failure

I INTRODUCTION

A. Definition. Congestive heart failure (CHF) occurs when the heart is unable to pump sufficient amounts of blood at normal filling pressures to meet the metabolic demands of the body.

B. Clinical manifestations classically include fatigue, dyspnea, orthopnea, paroxysmal nocturnal dyspnea (PND), weight gain, and peripheral edema.

C. Incidence. In the United States, CHF is common, affecting 1% of the general population and 10% of the population older than 75 years of age. CHF is now the most common hospital discharge diagnosis among patients older than 65 years. There are 400,000 new cases each year.

D. Mortality rates. The overall annual mortality rate for patients with CHF is 20%. For patients with severe CHF who have dyspnea at rest, the mortality rate is 50%. For those with pure diastolic dysfunction, the mortality rate is 8%.

II CLASSIFICATION. There are many different classification schemes. The most useful include the following:

A. Acute versus chronic onset

1. **Patients with acute CHF** in the setting of acute myocardial infarction (AMI) can be classified according to the **Killip classification system** (Table 16-1). The clinical and radiologic examination of the patient can determine the severity of heart failure and also the prognosis.

2. **Patients with chronic CHF** can be classified according to the **New York Heart Association (NYHA) functional classification system** (Table 16-2).

B. Left-sided versus right-sided failure. The distinction between left-sided and right-sided failure is based primarily on signs found during the physical examination.

1. **Left-sided failure**

   a. **Signs** of left-sided failure include:

      (1) **Rales**

      (2) **An abnormal left ventricular impulse** [i.e., a sustained or displaced point of maximal impulse (PMI)]

      (3) **A left-sided third heart sound (S$_3$)**

      (4) **Pulsus alternans** (i.e., an alternation between strong and weak peripheral arterial pulses)

TABLE 16-1. Killip Classification System

Class	Description	In-Hospital Mortality Rate
I	No signs of left ventricular dysfunction	< 10%
II	S$_3$ gallop or rales found in less than 50% of the lung fields	20%
III	Rales found in at least 50% of the lung fields	40%
IV	Cardiogenic shock with hypotension and pulmonary edema*; myocardial necrosis usually exceeds 40%	≥ 50%

S$_3$ = third heard sound.
*Acute papillary muscle rupture and ventricular septal defect should also be considered in patients with cardiogenic shock.

    b. Causes of left-sided failure include:
        (1) Myocardial disorders (e.g., those disorders that cause left ventricular systolic or diastolic dysfunction) [see II C]
        (2) Valvular disorders (e.g., aortic stenosis and aortic or mitral regurgitation)
  2. Right-sided failure
    a. Signs of right-sided failure include:
        (1) An elevated jugular venous pressure
        (2) An abnormal hepatojugular reflux
        (3) An abnormal right ventricular impulse
        (4) A right-sided S$_3$
        (5) Hepatomegaly

TABLE 16-2. New York Heart Association (NYHA) Functional Classification System

Class	Description	One-Year Mortality Rate
I	Symptomatic only with greater than normal physical activity	5%
II	Symptomatic during normal activity	10%
III	Symptomatic with minimal activity	20%
IV	Symptomatic at rest	30-40%

   (6) Ascites
   (7) Peripheral edema
 b. Causes of right-sided failure include:
  (1) Left-sided failure. Evidence of biventricular failure may be found during the physical examination because the most common cause of right-sided failure is left-sided failure.
  (2) Mitral stenosis
  (3) Pulmonary hypertension (primary or secondary) [see Chapter 24]
  (4) Right ventricular infarction (usually occurring in the setting of left ventricular inferior wall infarction)
   (5) Endocarditis of the tricuspid or pulmonary valve
   (6) Pericardial disease (e.g., tamponade, pericarditis)
C. Systolic versus diastolic dysfunction. Left ventricular failure can be either systolic or diastolic. This distinction is important because it affects treatment. Often, patients have both systolic and diastolic dysfunction.
 1. Systolic dysfunction means that the heart's contractility is compromised. It implies that the left ventricular ejection fraction (LVEF) is below normal (usually $\leq 40\%$). Causes of systolic dysfunction include:
  a. Coronary artery disease (CAD) with prior MI or ongoing myocardial ischemia
  b. "Burned out" hypertensive, restrictive, or valvular (aortic or mitral) heart disease. Initially, these disorders may lead to diastolic dysfunction, but with time the heart dilates and the LVEF decreases.
  c. Dilated cardiomyopathy (i.e., disorders of the myocardium that are not caused by CAD, hypertension, or valvular disease). Table 16-3 provides some of the causes of dilated cardiomyopathy.

TABLE 16-3. Common Causes of Dilated Cardiomyopathy

Myocarditis
Peripartum (see Chapter 28)
Pheochromocytoma
Hypothyroidism
Toxins (e.g., ethanol)
Drugs (e.g., cocaine and heroin)
Medications (e.g., anthracyclines)
High-output states (e.g., thyrotoxicosis, anemia, arteriovenous fistula, Paget's disease, chronic liver disease, beriberi)
Collagen vascular diseases (e.g., lupus erythematosus, polyarteritis nodosa, Churg-Strauss syndrome, systemic sclerosis)
Idiopathic

2. **Diastolic dysfunction** means that the heart has normal contractility, but its ability to relax and allow filling during diastole is compromised. Diastolic dysfunction accounts for approximately 50% of all cases of heart failure, and these
patients have a normal or hyperdynamic LVEF. Causes of
diastolic dysfunction include:
   a. **Ischemia**
   b. **Disorders that lead to left ventricular hypertrophy
   (LVH),** such as hypertension, aortic stenosis, or hypertrophic cardiomyopathy (Figure 16-1)
   c. **Restrictive cardiomyopathy,** which usually is caused by
   infiltrative diseases (e.g., hemochromatosis, amyloidosis,
   sarcoidosis, or scleroderma)

HOT **KEY**

CHF with a low LVEF = systolic dysfunction.
CHF with a normal or high LVEF = diastolic dysfunction.

III APPROACH TO THE PATIENT

A. Assess the patient's symptoms. Assign a Killip class for patients
with acute CHF and a NYHA class for patients with chronic
CHF.
B. On the basis of the patient's history, physical examination, and
chest radiographs (Figures 16-2 and 16-3), categorize the failure
as predominantly left-sided, right-sided, or biventricular.
   1. If the patient has left-sided CHF, check the LVEF to determine whether the dysfunction is predominantly systolic or
   diastolic. The LVEF can be assessed using an echocardiogram, multiple gated acquisition (MUGA) scan, or left ventriculogram during cardiac catheterization.
   2. If the patient has right-sided CHF, use an echocardiogram to
   exclude left-sided CHF, mitral stenosis, pulmonary hypertension, right ventricular dysfunction, and tricuspid or pulmonic valve disorders.

HOT **KEY**

An echocardiogram is the best initial imaging study to
evaluate the structure and function of the ventricles, valves, and
pericardium.

C. In a patient with known CHF whose symptoms have wors-
ened, identify what precipitated the CHF exacerbation (Table
16-4).

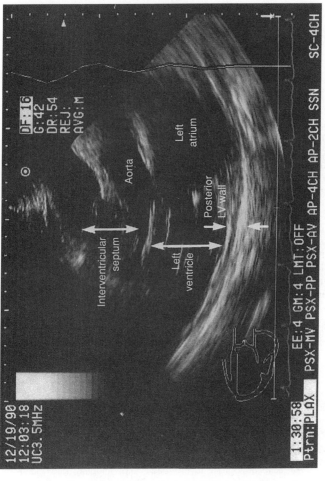

FIGURE 16-1. A two-dimensional echocardiogram showing hypertrophic cardiomyopathy. The severe thickening of the interventricular septum causes narrowing of the left ventricular outflow tract. (Reprinted with permission from Cheitlin MD, Sokolow M, McIlroy MB: *Clinical Cardiology*, 6th ed. Stamford, CT, Appleton & Lange, 1993, p 606.)

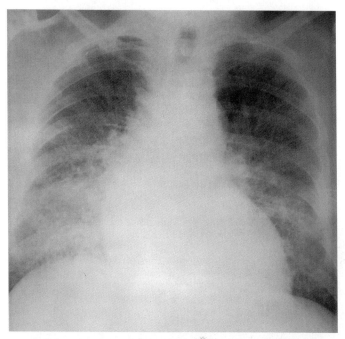

FIGURE 16-2. A posterior-anterior (PA) chest radiograph showing severe cardiomegaly and pulmonary edema, suggesting left-sided dysfunction and fluid overload. (Courtesy of C. Colangelo, M.D., San Francisco, CA)

IV TREATMENT

A. **Goals** of CHF therapy are twofold:
   1. **Reduce symptoms**
   2. **Reduce mortality**
B. **Acute CHF.** AMI is the most common cause of acute heart failure, leading to both systolic and diastolic dysfunction. Management of AMI is discussed in Chapter 13 V.
C. **Chronic systolic dysfunction**
   1. Aggressively treat the underlying cause of the CHF. For example, in patients with ischemic cardiomyopathy, consider revascularization with angioplasty or coronary artery bypass graft (CABG) surgery. In patients with aortic stenosis, perform valve replacement or valvuloplasty.
   2. Manage the symptoms and minimize the risk of complications from CHF.

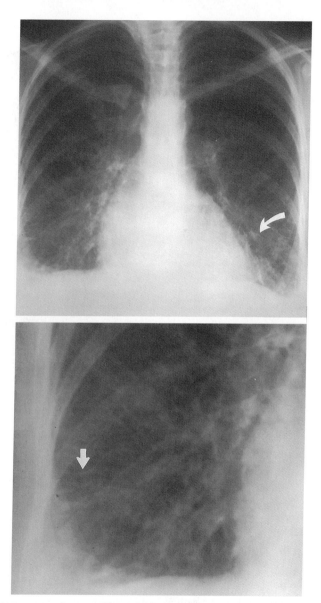

FIGURE 16-3. This patient has left-sided heart failure owing to chronic diastolic dysfunction caused by long-standing hypertension. (A) The long septal lines flanking the left border of the heart (*curved arrow*) represent Kerley A lines. (B) A magnified view of the right costophrenic sulcus (*straight arrow*) shows multiple Kerley B lines. (Courtesy of C. Colangelo, M.D., San Francisco, CA)

TABLE 16-4. Factors That Can Exacerbate Congestive Heart Failure

Myocardial ischemia or **infarction**
Arrhythmias, including brady- or tachyarrhythmias
Infections (e.g., endocarditis)
Upregulators (e.g., hyperthyroidism or pregnancy)
Medications, such as those agents that cause water retention
    [e.g., estrogens, steroids, nonsteroidal anti-inflammatory agents
    (NSAIDS)] or decrease contractility (e.g., β blockers, verapamil,
diltiazem, propafenone)
Noncompliance (e.g., forgetting to take medications or ignoring
    dietary restrictions)

  a. First-line therapy
     (1) Diet. A low-salt diet is primarily used to control fluid overload. For patients with mild CHF, sodium intake should be reduced to 3 g/day. For those with severe CHF, sodium intake should be reduced to less than 1.5 g/day.
     (2) Diuretics are prescribed to treat symptoms of fluid overload (e.g., rales, peripheral edema). They can reduce the incidence of CHF exacerbations, thus reducing the need for hospitalization.
       (a) In patients with mild CHF and normal renal function, hydrochlorothiazide or spironolactone (25 mg orally per day) may be all that is needed. Spironolactone has been shown to improve survival in CHF patients.
       (b) In patients with fluid overload, furosemide (20–80 mg orally once or twice daily) is commonly used.
       (c) If fluid overload becomes more severe, metolazone (2.5–5 mg orally per day) can be added to the furosemide.
     (3) Vasodilators
       (a) Angiotensin-converting enzyme (ACE) inhibitors are considered first-line therapy for patients with asymptomatic or symptomatic systolic dysfunction (see Appendix B). These agents have been shown to both reduce symptoms and mortality. Angiotensin receptor blockers (e.g., losartan) may be considered for patients who cannot tolerate ACE inhibitors.
       (b) Hydralazine and a long-acting nitrate can be added to ACE inhibitors if pulmonary congestion

or a low cardiac output (CO) persists, despite maximum doses of an ACE inhibitor. Alternatively, hydralazine and isosorbide dinitrate can be substituted for ACE inhibitors in patients with a contraindication to ACE inhibitors (e.g., hyperkalemia, severe renal insufficiency, bilateral renal artery stenosis, or angioedema).

(4) Digoxin has been shown to reduce symptoms of heart failure, but not to decrease mortality. Digoxin is generally recommended for patients who remain symptomatic despite other therapy (e.g., diuretics and vasodilators).

(5) Anticoagulation therapy (e.g., warfarin) is indicated for patients with CHF who have atrial fibrillation, left ventricular thrombus, systemic embolism, or a history of deep venous thrombosis.

b. Second-line therapy. Patients with severe CHF that is **refractory to general treatment measures** should be evaluated for more aggressive therapy.

(1) β Blockers may have a mortality benefit for patients with severe CHF. β-Blocker therapy (with metoprolol or carvedilol) should be started at a very low dose (i.e., 3.125–6.25 mg orally twice a day) in patients with well-compensated CHF.

(2) Dobutamine. Intravenous dopamine (2.5–5 μg/kg/min) and dobutamine (2.5–7.5 μg/kg/min) may be beneficial for patients with severe CHF that is refractory to standard outpatient treatment. This therapy, however, has not been shown to improve survival. Admission to the hospital (for 24–48 hours) is almost always necessary.

(3) Antiarrhythmic therapy. Forty percent of the mortality in patients with CHF is sudden, presumably due to ventricular tachycardia or fibrillation. Therefore, high-risk patients (e.g., survivors of ventricular tachycardia or fibrillation who have a reduced LVEF) may benefit from antiarrhythmic therapy. Controversy exists over whether this therapy should be used in lower-risk patients with nonsustained ventricular tachycardia.

(a) Amiodarone is the only antiarrhythmic medication that may provide a mortality benefit in high-risk patients with systolic dysfunction. Amiodarone should be used cautiously, however, because it can acutely exacerbate heart failure. Doses of digoxin and warfarin should be reduced by approximately 50% in patients being treated with amiodarone.

    (b) Automatic implantable cardioverter defibrillators (AICDs) should also be considered for high-risk patients and may be more effective than amiodarone therapy.

  (4) Heart transplantation can be considered for patients younger than 65 years with severe, irreversible CHF that is refractory to maximal medical therapy.

HOT

KEY

First- and second-generation calcium channel blockers should generally be avoided in patients with systolic dysfunction. Third-generation agents (e.g., amlodipine) have been shown to be safe in these patients, but should generally be used after β blocker and ACE inhibitor therapies have been maximized.

D. Chronic diastolic dysfunction
  1. General measures
    a. Diuretics should be titrated carefully to relieve congestive symptoms.
    b. Antihypertensive agents. β Blockers and calcium channel blockers are the drugs of choice to improve left ventricular relaxation.
    c. Atrial and ventricular pacing may improve ventricular filling in selected patients with bradycardia, long PR intervals, or both.

HOT

KEY

Digoxin and other inotropes should be avoided unless systolic dysfunction is also present.

---

  2. Specific management is aimed at the cause of the diastolic dysfunction.
    a. Ischemia. If the diastolic dysfunction is the result of ischemia, use antianginal therapy and revascularization with angioplasty or CABG when appropriate (see Chapter 14).
    b. Hypertension. If the diastolic dysfunction is the result of hypertensive heart disease, administer β blockers, calcium channel blockers, or ACE inhibitors.
    c. Aortic stenosis. If aortic stenosis is the cause of CHF, perform aortic valve replacement.
    d. Hypertrophic cardiomyopathy. β Blockers and calcium channel blockers are the first-line agents. Other measures include:

(1) Instructing patients to avoid strenuous physical activity
(2) Administering an antibiotic to prevent bacterial endocarditis
(3) Considering amiodarone for patients with ventricular arrhythmias despite aggressive β-blocker therapy
(4) Performing a septal myomectomy in patients with refractory symptoms
  e. Restrictive cardiomyopathy
(1) Diuretics and **nitrates** may be used to treat congestive symptoms.
(2) Cardiac transplantation is the only definitive treatment.

References
Baker DW, Konstam MA, Bottorff M, et al: Management of heart failure. Pharmacologic treatment. *JAMA* 272(17):1361–1366, 1994.
Gaasch WH: Diagnosis and treatment of heart failure based on left ventricular systolic or diastolic dysfunction. *JAMA* 271(16):1276–1280, 1994.
LeJemtel TH, Sonnenblick EH, Frishman WH: Diagnosis and management of heart failure. In *Hurst's The Heart,* 9th ed. Edited by Alexander RW, Schlant RC, Fuster V. New York, McGraw-Hill, 1998, pp 745–782.

PART V

VALVULAR HEART DISEASE

17. Aortic Valve Disease

I **INTRODUCTION.** The two major types of aortic valve disease are aortic stenosis and aortic regurgitation. Early recognition and treatment of these diseases can help prevent serious complications.

A. Incidence. As the population ages, the incidence of aortic stenosis and regurgitation increases.

B. Classification. Aortic valve disease can be classified as mild, moderate, or severe.

1. **The degree of aortic stenosis** is based on the aortic valve area (AVA), which is normally 3 cm^2. As the AVA decreases, the aortic stenosis becomes more severe (Table 17-1). The AVA can be assessed using echocardiography or during cardiac catheterization.

2. **The degree of aortic regurgitation** is based on the physical examination, echocardiogram, or aortogram during cardiac catheterization.

II **AORTIC STENOSIS**

A. Causes. Congenital or acquired disorders can cause aortic stenosis.

1. **Congenital causes.** Detection of aortic stenosis in patients younger than 30 years usually suggests a congenital etiology.

   a. Unicuspid or **bicuspid aortic valve disease** is found in 0.5%–2% of the population, and is a congenital abnormality that can lead to aortic stenosis. In patients between the ages of 40–60 years, calcification of the bicuspid aortic valve is a common cause of aortic stenosis.

   b. Subvalvular aortic stenosis is less common. This disorder can accompany hypertrophic cardiomyopathy or result from fibromuscular hypertrophy in the left ventricular outflow tract.

2. **Acquired causes**

   a. Rheumatic aortic stenosis. Aortic stenosis may be seen in association with mitral valve disease secondary to rheumatic heart disease.

TABLE 17-1. Classification of Aortic Stenosis	
Classification	Aortic Valve Area (cm^2)
Mild	> 1.2
Moderate	0.75–1.2
Severe	< 0.75
Critical	≤ 0.6

    b. Senile calcific aortic stenosis. Degenerative calcification of the aortic valve accounts for 90% of the need for aortic valve replacement in patients older than 70 years.

B. Approach to the patient

  1. Patient history. When the degree of aortic stenosis becomes hemodynamically significant (i.e., when the mean left ventricular-aortic pressure gradient is ≥ 30 mm Hg or the AVA is below 0.75 cm^2), symptoms may develop.

HOT KEY

The classic triad of symptoms related to aortic stenosis includes angina, syncope, and dyspnea.

    a. Angina is the most common symptom of aortic stenosis and results from the increased demand for oxygen in the left ventricle. Occasionally, patients will not report angina because they have already reduced their activity level to prevent it from occurring.

    b. Syncope can result from arrhythmias, myocardial ischemia, exercise-induced reflex vasodilation, or transient cerebral ischemia (usually occurring in elderly patients with coexisting cerebrovascular disease).

    c. Dyspnea usually indicates congestive heart failure (CHF). Other symptoms of CHF include orthopnea, fatigue, and pedal edema.

  2. Physical examination findings

    a. Evaluation of the carotid pulse. The intensity and upslope of the carotid pulse will diminish as the severity of aortic stenosis increases. The pulse is diminished and delayed (i.e., **pulsus parvus et tardus**).

    b. Palpation. Severe aortic stenosis will result in left ventricular hypertrophy (LVH), which can be detected by a diffuse or laterally displaced impulse over the apex. If a thrill is present, the aortic stenosis is usually severe.

c. Auscultation

   (1) Heart sounds. Severe aortic stenosis will result in a soft, delayed aortic component of the second heart sound (A_2). If aortic stenosis has caused pulmonary hypertension, the pulmonary component of the second heart sound (P_2) will be accentuated.

   (2) Murmurs

      (a) Classically, aortic stenosis is associated with a harsh **crescendo-decrescendo systolic murmur** that is heard loudest at the base of the heart and radiates to the carotid arteries.

      (b) As aortic stenosis becomes more severe, the peak of the murmur occurs later in systole.

      (c) Gallop. As LVH develops, a left ventricular fourth heart sound (S_4) will become evident. If left ventricular failure occurs, a third heart sound (S_3) may be appreciated.

3. Diagnostic tests. All patients should have a 12-lead electrocardiogram (ECG) and a chest radiograph. If cardiac symptoms are present or if severe aortic stenosis is suspected, further testing is indicated.

   a. ECG. An ECG is usually performed to detect LVH, left atrial abnormality (LAA), and conduction defects [ranging from first-degree atrioventricular (AV) block to left bundle branch block (LBBB)].

   b. Chest radiograph. Although the cardiac silhouette is usually normal, the heart will be enlarged in the late stages of left ventricular failure and dilatation. Aortic valve calcification may also be seen on the chest radiograph; however, it does not necessarily indicate aortic stenosis.

   c. Echocardiogram. A transthoracic Doppler echocardiogram is usually obtained to examine left ventricular systolic function, screen for congenital causes of aortic stenosis, quantify the extent of aortic valve dysfunction, and rule out multivalvular disease.

   d. Cardiac catheterization

      (1) For symptomatic patients who are candidates for aortic valve replacement (Table 17-2), quantification of the AVA and pressure gradient across the aortic valve can be determined during cardiac catheterization.

      (2) In addition, coronary angiography is generally performed in men older than 40 years and women older than 50 years to determine whether coronary artery bypass graft (CABG) surgery may also be needed at the time of aortic valve replacement.

C. Natural history. If aortic valve replacement is not performed, the prognosis will be determined by the patient's symptoms.

TABLE 17-2. Indications and Contraindications for Aortic Valve Replacement

Indications
Severe aortic valve disease (stenosis or regurgitation) with at least one of the following:
- Symptoms of angina, syncope, or dyspnea
- Left ventricular dilatation or systolic dysfunction
- Critical aortic stenosis (i.e., an AVA $\leq$ 0.6 cm^2 or a mean pressure gradient $\geq$ 60 mm Hg) in the absence of symptoms

Contraindications*
Comorbidities [e.g., severe COPD, terminal malignancy] that would place the patient at an unacceptably high risk for perioperative complications

AVA = aortic valve area; COPD = chronic obstructive pulmonary disease.
*Advanced age and a poor left ventricular ejection fraction (LVEF) are not contraindications to valve replacement.

1. For patients with angina, average survival is 5 years.
2. For patients with syncope, average survival is 3–4 years.
3. For patients with dyspnea (as a symptom of CHF), average survival is less than 2 years.

D. Complications

1. **Myocardial ischemia** or **infarction** can occur as the demand for myocardial oxygen becomes greater than the supply. Elderly patients with coexisting coronary artery disease (CAD) are at increased risk for this complication because CAD further decreases the oxygen supply.

2. **Ventricular arrhythmias** can result from LVH or myocardial ischemia. Annually, sudden death occurs in 3%–5% of patients who have asymptomatic aortic stenosis and in 15% of patients who have symptomatic aortic stenosis. This complication is rare in patients with chronic aortic regurgitation.

3. **Exertional syncope** that is not related to an arrhythmic disorder indicates a poor prognosis.

4. **CHF** is a late complication.

5. **Infective endocarditis** can also occur.

E. Treatment. The key to treating a patient with aortic stenosis is to determine whether the patient has symptoms.

1. **Aortic valve replacement** should be considered in patients with symptomatic aortic stenosis or critical asymptomatic aortic stenosis (i.e., an AVA $\leq$ 0.6 cm^2 or a mean pressure gradient $\geq$ 60 mm Hg).

2. **Antibiotic prophylaxis** should be used in all patients with aortic stenosis to prevent bacterial endocarditis (see Chapter 22).

3. **Aortic balloon valvuloplasty** can be used to increase the AVA (usually by 50%–70%); however, restenosis is very common. This procedure is generally reserved for elderly patients who are highly symptomatic and who have an unacceptably high risk for life-threatening complications with aortic valve replacement.

F. Follow-up
   1. **Asymptomatic patients** should receive a history and physical examination every 3–6 months and a Doppler echocardiogram every year. Patients should also be educated about the importance of immediately reporting symptoms and continuing antibiotic prophylaxis.
   2. **Symptomatic patients** should generally be referred for aortic valve replacement (see Table 17-2).

III Aortic Regurgitation

A. Causes. Aortic regurgitation is usually caused by disorders that affect the leaflets, the commissures, or the aortic root.
   1. Disorders that affect the aortic leaflets or commissures include:
      a. **Rheumatic heart disease**
      b. **Congenital bicuspid valve disease**
      c. **Myxomatous aortic valve degeneration**
      d. **Infective endocarditis**
   2. Disorders that affect the aortic root include:
      a. **Ascending aortic aneurysm** (e.g., hypertension, Marfan's syndrome, Reiter's syndrome, ankylosing spondylitis)
      b. **Ascending aortic dissection**
      c. **Trauma**
      d. **Aortitis** (e.g., syphilis, Takayasu's disease)

HOT **KEY** — The four main causes of acute aortic regurgitation are infective endocarditis, rheumatic fever, trauma, and acute aortic dissection.

B. Approach to the patient
   1. **Patient history**
      a. **Dyspnea,** fatigue, and pedal edema signify left ventricular failure.
      b. **Angina** can occur; however, it is unusual unless concomitant CAD exists.
      c. **Neck pulsations** and a forceful heartbeat are common because of the large stroke volume that occurs with aortic regurgitation.

2. **Physical examination findings**
   a. **Evaluation of vital signs.** A widened pulse pressure is a classic finding when aortic regurgitation becomes hemodynamically significant. If the patient's diastolic pressure is greater than 70 mm Hg, aortic regurgitation is usually mild or moderate.
   b. **Evaluation of the pulse.** The diagnosis of severe aortic regurgitation can be made based on the pulse alone (Table 17-3).
   c. **Palpation.** If the left ventricle is dilated, the apical impulse will be laterally displaced. A left ventricular heave and a diastolic thrill usually signify severe aortic regurgitation.
   d. **Auscultation**
      (1) **Heart sounds.** Severe aortic regurgitation will result in a soft first heart sound (S_1). Rapid ventricular filling in diastole may restrict the opening of the anterior mitral leaflet, resulting in a soft mitral closure sound.
      (2) **Murmurs** of aortic regurgitation are best appreciated while the patient is sitting upright and holding her breath at end-expiration.
         (a) Aortic regurgitation classically produces a high-pitched, decrescendo, blowing, diastolic murmur along the left sternal border.
         (b) With severe aortic regurgitation, rapid left ventricular filling in diastole may cause the anterior leaflet of the mitral valve to vibrate, resulting in the diastolic murmur known as the **Austin Flint rumble.**

TABLE 17-3. Pulses That Indicate Severe Aortic Regurgitation

Pulse	Description
Corrigan's pulse (i.e., water-hammer pulse)	A peripheral pulse that has a rapid upstroke, followed by a sudden collapse
de Musset's sign	A bobbing movement of the head occurring with each cardiac impulse
Duroziez's sign	A systolic and diastolic bruit heard over the femoral artery
Müller's sign	The rhythmic pulsation of the uvula
Quincke's pulse	Arterial pulsations observed in the nail bed

        (3) Gallop. Because of rapid left ventricular filling in diastole, an S_3 may be appreciated.

  3. Diagnostic tests. The following approach to diagnostic testing is recommended for patients with suspected aortic regurgitation.

    a. ECG. As with aortic stenosis, an ECG often shows LVH, LAA, and conduction defects.

    b. Chest radiograph

      (1) In patients with chronic aortic regurgitation, left ventricular dilatation is the most common finding.

      (2) In patients with acute aortic regurgitation, the heart size may be normal.

    c. Blood cultures. If endocarditis is suspected, 2-3 sets of blood cultures should be obtained.

    d. Echocardiogram

      (1) A **transthoracic Doppler echocardiogram** is useful for measuring left ventricular size and systolic function, evaluating the structure of the aortic valve, looking for vegetations, measuring the aortic root, and estimating the severity of aortic regurgitation.

      (2) A **transesophageal echocardiogram** is often useful for evaluating patients with suspected endocarditis or aortic dissection.

    e. Cardiac catheterization

      (1) Aortography can be used to determine the severity of aortic regurgitation.

      (2) Coronary angiography is performed in patients being considered for aortic valve replacement who are at risk for concomitant CAD.

C. Natural history

  1. For patients with mild or moderate aortic regurgitation, roughly 90% will survive for 10 years if the regurgitation is left untreated. For those with severe aortic regurgitation, only 50% will survive 10 years.

  2. If CHF develops, the prognosis rapidly worsens to less than 2 years survival without aortic valve replacement.

D. Complications are similar for patients with aortic regurgitation or aortic stenosis (see II D).

E. Treatment depends on whether the onset of disease is chronic or acute.

  1. Chronic aortic regurgitation

    a. Aortic valve replacement (see Table 17-2) should be offered to patients with severe chronic aortic regurgitation and evidence of an impaired left ventricular ejection fraction (LVEF).

    b. Medical therapy

      (1) Vasodilators. For patients with at least moderate

aortic regurgitation, **angiotensin-converting enzyme (ACE) inhibitors** are indicated to attenuate left ventricular dilatation and failure.

   (2) Antibiotic prophylaxis should be used to prevent bacterial endocarditis (see Chapter 22).

2. Acute aortic regurgitation is considered a surgical emergency. Patients usually present with acute pulmonary edema and poor cardiac output (CO).

   a. Aortic valve replacement should be performed immediately in patients with hemodynamically severe acute aortic regurgitation and pulmonary edema. If acute endocarditis is also present, antibiotics should be administered before aortic valve replacement.

   b. Medical therapy includes intravenous nitroprusside for afterload reduction, diuretics for pulmonary edema, and vasopressors (e.g., dopamine) for hypotension. Hemodynamic monitoring with a pulmonary artery (PA) catheter is usually indicated.

F. Follow-up is the same as for aortic stenosis (see II E).

References

Carabello BA, Crawford FA: Valvular heart disease. *N Engl J Med* 337(1):32–41, 1997.

O'Rourke RA: Aortic valve stenosis: a common clinical entity. *Curr Probl Cardiol* 23(8):434–471, 1998.

Rahimtoola SH: Aortic valve disease. In *Hurst's The Heart,* 9th ed. Edited by Alexander RW, Schlant RC, Fuster V. New York, McGraw-Hill, 1998, pp 1759–1788.

18. Mitral Valve Disease

I   **INTRODUCTION.** The three major types of mitral valve disease are mitral stenosis, mitral regurgitation, and mitral valve prolapse (MVP). MVP is a billowing of the mitral leaflets into the left atrium during systole. Prompt diagnosis and assessment of these diseases can decrease the likelihood of serious complications.

A. **Incidence**
   1. **Clinically significant mitral stenosis** or **regurgitation** occurs in less than 5% of the general population. Mitral stenosis often presents in young adulthood, while mitral regurgitation is typically seen in older patients.
   2. **MVP** occurs in approximately 5%-10% of the general population and is more common in women. MVP is not usually associated with serious complications.

B. **Classification.** Mitral valve diseases can be classified as mild, moderate, or severe.
   1. The **degree of mitral stenosis** is based on the mitral valve area (MVA), which is normally 4–6 cm^2. As the MVA decreases, mitral stenosis becomes more severe (Table 18-1). The MVA can be assessed using echocardiography or during cardiac catheterization.
   2. The **degree of mitral regurgitation and MVP** is based primarily on findings of the physical examination, echocardiogram, and left ventriculogram during cardiac catheterization.

TABLE 18-1. Classification of Mitral Stenosis

Classification	Mitral Valve Area (cm^2)
Mild	> 2.0
Moderate	1.0–2.0
Severe	< 1.0

HOT KEY

Tumors (e.g., a left atrial myxoma) should be excluded if other causes of mitral stenosis are not found.

▐▐ MITRAL STENOSIS

A. Causes

1. **Rheumatic heart disease,** which leads to scarring, calcification, and contraction of the mitral leaflets and chordae tendineae, is the most common cause of mitral stenosis (Figure 18-1). After the initial attack of rheumatic fever, it typically takes 5–20 years for mitral stenosis to become hemodynamically significant.

2. **Rarer causes** include:

    a. Severe mitral annular calcification

    b. Chronic valvulitis (resulting from systemic lupus erythematosus, amyloid, or carcinoid syndrome)

B. Approach to the patient

1. **Patient history.** Classically, patients with mitral stenosis remain asymptomatic for many years, even though the severity of the disease is gradually worsening. However, when the left atrial pressure becomes chronically elevated (leading to increased pressure in the pulmonary vasculature and right ventricle), symptoms will develop.

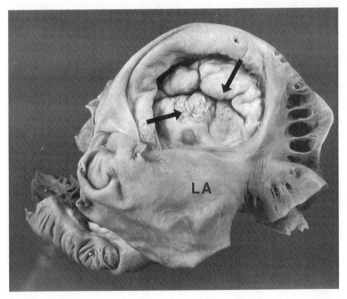

FIGURE 18-1. Looking down from the dilated left atrium (*LA*), the mitral leaflets (*arrows*) have been distorted as a result of the effects of rheumatic heart disease. The fibrosis and calcification cause leaflet immobility and severe mitral stenosis. (Courtesy of P.C. Ursell, M.D., San Francisco, CA)

    a. Dyspnea on exertion is the most common symptom of mitral stenosis.

    b. Chest pain may occur as a result of pulmonary hypertension and right ventricular ischemia.

    c. Hemoptysis may occur as a result of rupturing of the pulmonary capillaries or bronchial veins.

    d. Hoarseness may occasionally develop as the recurrent laryngeal nerve becomes compressed by the enlarged left atrium or pulmonary artery.

2. Physical examination findings

    a. Palpation. If a right ventricular lift, palpable pulmonary artery, and a diastolic thrill are appreciated, severe mitral stenosis with right ventricular failure can be diagnosed.

    b. Auscultation is the key to diagnosing mitral stenosis.

      (1) Heart sounds

        (a) The first heart sound (S_1) is loud.

        (b) The mitral opening snap is best heard along the left sternal border and occurs shortly after the second heart sound (S_2). As the severity of mitral stenosis increases, the opening snap moves closer to the S_2.

        (c) If mitral stenosis has led to pulmonary hypertension, the pulmonary component of the second heart sound (P_2) will be accentuated.

      (2) Murmurs. A low-pitched diastolic rumble is heard, and is most prominent at the apex.

      (3) Gallop. A right-sided third heart sound (S_3) or fourth heart sound (S_4) may indicate right ventricular dysfunction.

    c. Abdominal examination. Hepatomegaly and ascites indicate hepatic congestion.

    d. Peripheral examination. Pedal edema and cyanosis indicate right ventricular failure and low cardiac output (CO), respectively.

3. Diagnostic tests. All patients should have a 12-lead electrocardiogram (ECG) and a chest radiograph. Further diagnostic testing is indicated for patients who have cardiac symptoms or if severe mitral stenosis is suspected.

    a. ECG

      (1) Atrial fibrillation is a common complication of mitral stenosis. The ECG, however, may show left atrial abnormality (LAA) in patients with sinus rhythm.

      (2) If pulmonary hypertension is present, the ECG may show right axis deviation (RAD), right ventricular hypertrophy (RVH), or right bundle branch block (RBBB).

   b. Chest radiograph. Left atrial enlargement, pulmonary
      vascular congestion, prominent pulmonary arteries, or
      right ventricular enlargement may be seen.

HOT
▶
KEY

Kerley B lines (i.e., linear shadows on the chest radiograph
that are perpendicular to the pleura at the base of the lungs)
are the result of fibrosis and lymphatic engorgement caused by
chronic pulmonary hypertension (see Figure 16-3).

---

   c. Echocardiogram
      (1) A **transthoracic echocardiogram** can show restricted
         mitral leaflet motion and left atrial enlargement.
      (2) A **Doppler echocardiogram** can be used to measure
         the diastolic pressure gradient across the mitral valve
         and to calculate the MVA.
   d. Cardiac catheterization may be performed in sympto-
      matic patients who are candidates for mitral balloon
      valvotomy or surgical mitral valve replacement.
      (1) Cardiac catheterization is used to measure the dias-
         tolic pressure gradient across the mitral valve [i.e., by
         simultaneously measuring the left ventricular pres-
         sure and the pulmonary capillary wedge pressure
         (PCWP)] and to calculate the MVA. The PCWP is
         used to estimate the left atrial pressure.
      (2) Coronary angiography is usually performed in men
         older than 40 years and women older than 50 years
         to identify any need for coronary artery bypass
         graft (CABG) surgery at the time of mitral valve
         replacement.
C. Natural history. For those patients with severe mitral stenosis
   who do not undergo mitral valve replacement, the prognosis depends on the severity of their symptoms.
   1. For **asymptomatic patients,** the 10-year survival rate is
      greater than 60%.
   2. For patients with **dyspnea on minimal exertion,** the 10-year
      survival rate is less than 40%.
   3. For patients with **dyspnea at rest,** the 5-year survival rate
      without mitral valve replacement is less than 15%.
D. Complications
   1. Atrial fibrillation develops in more than 50% of patients
      with severe mitral stenosis. For those patients with atrial fib-
      rillation who do not receive anticoagulation therapy, the rate
      of thromboembolism is as high as 20% per year.
   2. Pulmonary hypertension with **right ventricular failure** can
      develop.

    3. Severe tricuspid regurgitation can occur and does not always resolve after mitral valve replacement.

    4. Infective endocarditis can also occur.

E. Treatment

    1. Mitral balloon valvotomy is the treatment of choice in most patients with symptomatic mitral stenosis. This procedure is performed in the cardiac catheterization laboratory and involves inflating a balloon that has been inserted into the mitral valve to increase the MVA. Contraindications include:

        a. Left atrial thrombus

        b. Severe mitral valve calcification and rigidity

        c. Severe subvalvular disease (which can be assessed using echocardiography)

    2. Mitral valve replacement is appropriate for patients with symptomatic mitral stenosis who are not candidates for balloon valvotomy.

    3. Antibiotic prophylaxis is recommended for all patients with mitral stenosis to prevent infective endocarditis (see Chapter 22).

F. Follow-up

    1. Asymptomatic patients should receive a history and physical examination every 6 months and a Doppler echocardiogram every year. Patients should be educated about the importance of immediately reporting symptoms and continuing antibiotic prophylaxis.

    2. Patients with cardiac symptoms should generally receive closer follow-up.

III MITRAL REGURGITATION

A. Causes. Normal systolic valve closure requires proper functioning of the mitral valve annulus, valve leaflets, chordae tendineae, papillary muscles, and left ventricular myocardium. Therefore, disorders affecting any of those structures can result in mitral regurgitation.

    1. Disorders affecting the mitral valve annulus include:

        a. Left ventricular dilatation of any etiology (e.g., cardiomyopathy, aortic insufficiency)

        b. Calcification of the mitral annulus

    2. Disorders affecting the mitral valve leaflets include:

        a. Rheumatic heart disease

        b. MVP

        c. Infective endocarditis

        d. Connective tissue diseases (e.g., Marfan's syndrome, Ehlers-Danlos syndrome)

        e. Collagen vascular diseases (e.g., systemic lupus erythematosus)

    3. Disorders that cause the chordae tendineae to rupture include:

      a. Degenerative myxomatous

      b. Trauma

      c. Infective endocarditis

    4. Disorders that cause dysfunction or rupture of the papillary muscles include:

      a. Myocardial ischemia or infarction

      b. Trauma

    5. Disorders affecting the left ventricular myocardium include:

      a. Coronary artery disease (CAD)

      b. Dilated cardiomyopathy

      c. Hypertrophic cardiomyopathy

B. Approach to the patient

    1. Patient history

      a. For patients with **chronic mitral regurgitation,** dyspnea and fatigue are common initial symptoms. Orthopnea, paroxysmal nocturnal dyspnea (PND), and peripheral edema may also be present.

      b. For patients with **acute mitral regurgitation** (usually resulting from rupture of the chordae tendineae, or rupture or dysfunction of the papillary muscle), sudden and severe symptoms related to congestive heart failure (CHF) [e.g., flash pulmonary edema] are common.

    2. Physical examination findings

      a. Palpation. Severe mitral regurgitation is usually associated with a left ventricular lift, a laterally displaced apical impulse, and a systolic thrill.

      b. Auscultation

        (1) Heart sounds. The S_1 will be diminished and the S_2 will be widely split.

        (2) Murmurs. A high-pitched holosystolic murmur is heard at the apex and radiates to the left axilla.

        (3) Gallop

          (a) A left-sided S_3 may be heard when mitral regurgitation becomes hemodynamically significant.

          (b) A left-sided S_4 may be heard with acute mitral regurgitation.

          (c) Right-sided gallops may be appreciated when right ventricular dysfunction is present.

      c. Abdominal examination. Hepatomegaly and ascites indicate hepatic congestion.

      d. Peripheral examination. Pedal edema and cyanosis are related to right ventricular failure and a low CO, respectively.

    3. Diagnostic tests. As with mitral stenosis, all patients should have an ECG and a chest radiograph. If cardiac symptoms are present or if severe mitral regurgitation is suspected, further testing should be performed.

    a. ECG. LAA and left ventricular hypertrophy (LVH) may be seen with chronic mitral regurgitation.

    b. Chest radiograph. The left atrium and ventricle may be enlarged with chronic mitral regurgitation. Pulmonary edema may be seen with mitral regurgitation.

    c. Blood cultures. If endocarditis is suspected, 2–3 sets of blood cultures should be obtained.

    d. Echocardiogram. A transthoracic echocardiogram can be used to identify the cause and severity of mitral regurgitation, and to determine the degree of left ventricular dysfunction.

    e. Cardiac catheterization

        (1) Measurement of the left and right ventricular pressure can help determine the degree of ventricular dysfunction.

        (2) Left ventriculography can be used to assess the severity of mitral regurgitation and the left ventricular ejection fraction (LVEF).

        (3) Coronary angiography is usually recommended for patients who are at risk for CAD.

HOT **KEY**   A large *v* wave on the PCWP tracing often indicates severe mitral regurgitation. However, because this finding also occurs with CHF and ventricular septal defect, further testing is necessary to confirm the diagnosis.

C. Natural history. If the patient does not undergo treatment, his prognosis will generally depend on the severity of his symptoms and the degree of left ventricular dysfunction. Survival rates are comparable to those of patients with aortic regurgitation (see Chapter 17 III C).

D. Complications

    1. Atrial fibrillation develops in 10%-20% of patients with severe mitral regurgitation.

    2. Left ventricular dysfunction may develop as the LVEF decreases.

    3. Infective endocarditis can also occur.

E. Treatment

    1. Mitral valve surgery is the primary treatment option for patients with symptomatic mitral regurgitation.

HOT **KEY**   Because the LVEF may decline after mitral valve surgery, referral for mitral valve replacement should be made before the LVEF falls below approximately 50% in patients with severe mitral regurgitation.

---

   a. Mitral valve repair and placement of an **annuloplasty ring**
   may be performed in patients with noncalcified mitral
   valves. This therapy is preferred over valve replacement
   because it has fewer complications and the patient does
   not need anticoagulation therapy.
   b. Mitral valve replacement is an excellent option for patients
   with symptomatic mitral regurgitation who are not candidates for valve repair. Overall, patients with severe mitral
   regurgitation who undergo valve replacement will have an
   80% 5-year survival rate and a 60% 10-year survival rate.
   2. Medical therapy
   a. Angiotensin-converting enzyme (ACE) inhibitors may be
   used in patients with a low LVEF who are not eligible for
   valve surgery. These agents have been shown to reduce
   regurgitant volume.
   b. Digoxin and **diuretics** may also be added in patients with
   symptomatic CHF.
   c. Antibiotic prophylaxis should be used in all patients to
   prevent infective endocarditis (see Chapter 22).
F. Follow-up is the same as for patients with mitral stenosis (see II F).

IV MITRAL VALVE PROLAPSE

A. Causes. MVP may be caused by **disorders affecting the mitral
leaflets or chordae tendineae,** or an **underlying cardiac disorder**.
In some cases, the cause is unknown.
   1. Disorders affecting the mitral leaflets or chordae tendineae
   include:
   a. Familial disorders
   b. Connective tissue diseases (e.g., Marfan's syndrome,
   Ehlers-Danlos syndrome)
   2. Underlying cardiac disorders that can cause MVP include:
   a. CAD
   b. Rheumatic heart disease
   c. Cardiomyopathy (e.g., hypertrophic or dilated cardiomyopathy)
   3. Normal variant is the most common cause of MVP.
B. Approach to the patient. MVP is most commonly diagnosed in-
cidentally in asymptomatic patients during auscultation or with
echocardiography.
   1. Patient history. Symptoms, when present, usually include
   palpitations (the most common symptom), chest pain, dyspnea, and fatigue.
   2. Physical examination findings
   a. Skeletal examination. Evaluate the patient for scoliosis,
   pectus excavatum, and a narrowed anterior–posterior
   (AP) chest diameter.

   b. Auscultation. A high-pitched **midsystolic click** is a typical
      finding. The clicking sound is produced by sudden tensing
      of the mitral valve apparatus as the leaflets prolapse into
      the left atrium.
 3. **Diagnostic tests.** The following tests may be considered in
    the diagnostic evaluation.
    a. ECG. Nonspecific ST/T wave changes, a prolonged QT
       interval, and rhythm disturbances [e.g., premature atrial
       and ventricular complexes, paroxysmal supraventricular
       tachycardia (PSVT)] may be seen with MVP. An **ambula-
       tory Holter monitor** may be indicated for symptomatic
       patients.
    b. Chest radiograph. The cardiac silhouette is usually nor-
       mal; however, chest wall abnormalities (e.g., pectus exca-
       vatum) may be seen.
    c. An **echocardiogram** can be used to determine whether
       one or both of the mitral leaflets are prolapsing into the
       left atrium. This diagnostic test can also be used to assess
       the LVEF and to determine whether the patient has mi-
       tral regurgitation.
    d. Cardiac catheterization is rarely used in the diagnosis or
       assessment of MVP. When it is used, left ventriculography
       can confirm the diagnosis, assess the LVEF, and deter-
       mine whether the patient has mitral regurgitation.
C. Natural history. For most patients with MVP, the prognosis is
   good. However, if mitral regurgitation is also present, the risk
   for CHF increases.
D. Complications
 1. **Mitral regurgitation** may develop acutely (e.g., due to rup-
    tured chordae tendineae) or chronically (e.g., due to myxo-
    matous prolapsing leaflets).
 2. **Supraventricular tachycardia** is more common in patients
    with MVP compared to patients without MVP.
 3. **Sudden death** is an infrequent complication.
 4. **Thromboembolism** is more common in those with MVP.
 5. **Infective endocarditis** may occur in patients with both MVP
    and mitral regurgitation.
 6. **CHF** may occur as a late complication, usually in patients
    with MVP and mitral regurgitation.
E. Treatment
 1. **Antibiotic prophylaxis** should be used in patients with both
    MVP and mitral regurgitation to prevent bacterial endo-
    carditis. Patients with isolated MVP have a lower risk of en-
    docarditis and, therefore, do not need prophylaxis.
 2. **Dietary restrictions** (e.g., avoiding caffeine, alcohol, and to-
    bacco) and **β blockers** may be useful in patients with persis-
    tent palpitations.

F. Follow-up

1. **Asymptomatic patients** with isolated MVP should be assessed every 2 years. An echocardiogram may be considered every 5 years to screen for mitral regurgitation and left ventricular dysfunction.

2. **High-risk patients** with mitral regurgitation or left ventricular dysfunction should be followed more closely.

References

Bruce CJ, Nishimura RA: Clinical assessment and management of mitral stenosis. *Cardiol Clinics* 16(3):375–403, 1998.

Carabello BA, Crawford FA: Valvular heart disease. *N Engl J Med* 337(1):32–41, 1997.

Rahimtoola SH, Enriquez-Sarano M, Schaff HV, et al: Mitral valve disease. In *Hurst's The Heart,* 9th ed. Edited by Alexander RW, Schlant RC, Fuster V. New York, Mc-Graw-Hill, 1998, pp 1789–1820.

19. Pulmonic and Tricuspid Valve Disease

I INTRODUCTION

A. Pulmonic and tricuspid stenosis occur rarely. Pulmonic and tricuspid valvular insufficiency most commonly result from pulmonary hypertension.

B. Although pulmonic and tricuspid valve diseases are not usually life-threatening, appropriate management of patients with these diseases can help reduce the symptoms of right-sided heart failure and the incidence of bacterial endocarditis.

II PULMONIC VALVE DISEASES

A. Pulmonic stenosis

  1. Causes. Pulmonic stenosis is most commonly congenital in origin. Other causes include:
   a. Large vegetations
   b. Tumors
   c. Carcinoid syndrome

  2. Approach to the patient
   a. Patient history. Patients with pulmonic stenosis may develop symptoms of right-sided heart failure, which include fatigue and peripheral edema. As the right atrial pressure increases, gastrointestinal symptoms (e.g., anorexia and right upper quadrant pain from hepatomegaly) may also develop.

HOT KEY If carcinoid syndrome is the cause of pulmonic stenosis, the patient may experience symptoms of facial flushing, diarrhea, and wheezing.

---

   b. Physical examination findings
    (1) Examination of the internal jugular veins. If the internal jugular veins are distended, the patient has an elevated central venous pressure (CVP).
    (2) Palpation. A right ventricular lift indicates right ventricular dysfunction.
    (3) Auscultation
     (a) Heart sounds. If pulmonary hypertension is pres-

ent, the pulmonary component of the second
heart sound (P_2) will be accentuated.

    (b) Murmurs associated with pulmonic stenosis are
often difficult to appreciate.

  c. Diagnostic tests. All patients should have a 12-lead electrocardiogram (ECG) and a chest radiograph. Further
testing may be indicated if the patient has symptoms and
if severe pulmonic stenosis is suspected.

    (1) ECG. Right ventricular hypertrophy (RVH) and
right atrial enlargement may be seen.

    (2) Echocardiogram

      (a) A **transthoracic echocardiogram** can be used to
identify structural abnormalities in the pulmonic
valve.

      (b) A **Doppler echocardiogram** can be used to mea-
sure the pressure gradient across the pulmonic
valve, thereby estimating the pulmonic valve area.

    (3) Cardiac catheterization. Simultaneous recording of
the pressures from the right ventricle and the pulmonary artery can determine the pulmonic valve
pressure gradient.

3. Treatment. As with aortic and mitral valve diseases, treatment will depend on the severity of the patient's symptoms.
It is important to identify and treat the underlying cause of
the valvular abnormality.

  a. Balloon valvuloplasty is often used to treat severe pulmonic stenosis caused by a congenital disorder.

  b. Pulmonic valve replacement may be used to treat severe
pulmonic stenosis caused by acquired disorders (e.g., endocarditis, carcinoid syndrome) and to reduce the symptoms of right ventricular failure.

B. Pulmonic insufficiency

1. Causes. Pulmonic insufficiency is caused by pulmonic leaflet
or commissure diseases, or disorders that cause dilatation of
the pulmonic annulus.

  a. Pulmonic leaflet or commissure diseases include:

    (1) Infective endocarditis, the most common cause of
acute pulmonic insufficiency

    (2) Rheumatic heart disease

    (3) Congenital valve deformities

  b. Disorders that cause dilatation of the pulmonic annulus
include:

    (1) Pulmonary hypertension, the most common cause of
chronic pulmonic insufficiency

    (2) Pulmonary artery dilatation (e.g., Marfan's syn-
drome, syphilis)

2. Approach to the patient

  a. Patient history. In general, patients with isolated pulmonic insufficiency do not have symptoms. If pulmonary hypertension is also present, however, dyspnea, peripheral edema, and fatigue may be present.

b. Physical examination findings

    (1) Examination of the internal jugular veins can help determine whether the CVP is elevated.

    (2) Palpation may reveal a right ventricular lift.

    (3) Auscultation

        (a) Heart sounds. If pulmonary hypertension is present, the P_2 will be accentuated.

        (b) Murmurs. Pulmonic insufficiency is associated with a high-pitched diastolic decrescendo murmur along the left sternal border. This murmur is often difficult to distinguish from the murmur associated with aortic regurgitation.

c. Diagnostic tests

    (1) ECG. RVH and right atrial enlargement may be seen.

    (2) Blood cultures. If endocarditis is suspected, blood cultures should be obtained.

    (3) Echocardiogram

        (a) A **transthoracic echocardiogram** can be used to identify structural abnormalities and vegetations in the pulmonic valve and to measure right atrial and ventricular size.

        (b) A **Doppler echocardiogram** can be used to estimate the severity of pulmonic insufficiency and to measure pulmonary artery pressures.

    (4) Cardiac catheterization. Pulmonic insufficiency can be demonstrated by using pulmonary angiography. Right ventriculography can show pulmonary artery dilatation, assess the degree of systolic dysfunction, and measure ventricular size. Pulmonary artery pressures can be measured.

3. Treatment

    a. Because pulmonic insufficiency is generally well tolerated, only patients with pulmonary hypertension and right ventricular failure need treatment. Treatment of pulmonary hypertension is discussed in Chapter 24 V.

    b. Pulmonic valve replacement may be used to treat primary valve disorders.

III TRICUSPID VALVE DISEASES

A. Tricuspid stenosis

    1. Causes

        a. Rheumatic heart disease is the most common cause of tricuspid stenosis.

        b. Tumors (e.g., a right atrial myxoma; metastases from the kidneys, testicles, thyroid, liver, or skin) can cause tricuspid valve obstruction.

2. Approach to the patient

  a. Patient history. Patients with isolated tricuspid stenosis most commonly report dyspnea, peripheral edema, gastrointestinal symptoms, and fatigue.

  b. Physical examination findings

   (1) Examination of the internal jugular veins can be used to determine whether the CVP is elevated. A prominent *a* wave indicates impaired right ventricular filling with each atrial contraction.

   (2) Auscultation. A soft-pitched diastolic murmur along the left lower sternal border may be appreciated in patients with tricuspid stenosis.

  c. Diagnostic tests

   (1) ECG. Typically, the ECG will show a large upright P wave in lead II, which indicates right atrial enlargement. Criteria for RVH will be absent.

   (2) Echocardiogram

    (a) A **transthoracic echocardiogram** can demonstrate tricuspid valve fibrosis or calcification. It also can be used to identify masses that are obstructing the tricuspid valve (e.g., thrombi, vegetations, tumors).

    (b) A **Doppler echocardiogram** can be used to estimate the tricuspid valve area by measuring the diastolic pressure gradient across the tricuspid valve.

   (3) Cardiac catheterization. In symptomatic patients who are suitable candidates for tricuspid valve surgery, simultaneous recording of the pressures from the right atrium and the right ventricle can determine the tricuspid valve pressure gradient.

3. Treatment

  a. Diuretics and vasodilators (e.g., nitrates) may decrease the symptoms of venous congestion.

  b. Tricuspid valve replacement is often performed in patients with concomitant left-sided valve disease.

  c. Balloon valvuloplasty is an alternative to tricuspid valve replacement.

  d. Surgical debulking should be considered in patients who have a tumor obstructing the tricuspid valve.

B. Tricuspid regurgitation

1. Causes. Tricuspid regurgitation is caused by tricuspid leaflet or commissure diseases or by disorders that cause dilatation of the tricuspid annulus.

  a. Tricuspid leaflet or commissure diseases include:

      (1) Rheumatic heart disease
      (2) Myxomatous tricuspid valve degeneration
      (3) Tricuspid valve prolapse
      (4) Infective endocarditis
      (5) Congenital tricuspid valve disorders (e.g., Ebstein's anomaly)
      (6) Right atrial myxoma

  b. Disorders that cause dilatation of the tricuspid annulus are the most common causes of tricuspid regurgitation and include:

      (1) Right ventricular dysfunction (e.g., cardiomyopathy, right ventricular infarction or ischemia)
      (2) Pulmonary hypertension
      (3) Trauma

2. Approach to the patient

  a. Patient history. Because tricuspid regurgitation often accompanies right ventricular dysfunction or mitral stenosis, symptoms may include dyspnea, orthopnea, gastrointestinal symptoms, and pedal edema. If endocarditis is present, fever and fatigue may be present.

  b. Physical examination findings

      (1) Examination of the internal jugular veins may help to determine if the CVP is elevated. The characteristic *cv* wave is produced by the regurgitant flow into the right atrium and neck veins.

      (2) Auscultation. A holosystolic murmur at the left sternal border may be appreciated. As opposed to the murmur of mitral regurgitation, the murmur of tricuspid regurgitation **increases** with inspiration, as a result of increased venous return to the right side of the heart.

  c. Diagnostic tests

      (1) ECG. Because right ventricular dysfunction is common, the ECG may show right bundle branch block (RBBB), RVH, or both.

HOT **KEY** Atrial fibrillation is common in patients with severe tricuspid regurgitation.

---

      (2) Blood cultures. If endocarditis is suspected, blood cultures should be obtained.
      (3) Echocardiogram
        (a) A **transthoracic echocardiogram** can be used to accurately measure right atrial and ventricular

size. Tricuspid valve vegetations, prolapse, or chordae tendineae rupture may be revealed on the echocardiogram.

    (b) A **Doppler echocardiogram** can estimate the severity of tricuspid regurgitation and the degree of pulmonary hypertension.

(4) Cardiac catheterization

    (a) Right heart catheterization is an important diagnostic test used to document the severity of pulmonary hypertension. A prominent *cv* wave on the right atrial pressure tracing suggests severe tricuspid regurgitation.

    (b) Right ventriculography can provide angiographic evidence of tricuspid regurgitation.

3. Treatment

    a. Diuretics and vasodilators may be useful for patients with severe tricuspid regurgitation. If pulmonary hypertension is present, treatment should focus on reducing pulmonary pressures (see Chapter 24 V).

    b. Tricuspid valve repair (e.g., annuloplasty) **or replacement** may be indicated in patients with severe tricuspid regurgitation that is refractory to medical therapy.

References

Ewy GA: Tricuspid valve disease. In *Cardiology: physiology, pharmacology, diagnosis.* Edited by Parmley WW, Chatterjee K. New York: Lippincott, 1992, pp 1–19.

O'Rourke RA, Rackley CE, Edwards JE, et al: Tricuspid valve, pulmonic valve, and multivalvular disease. In *Hurst's The Heart,* 9th ed. Edited by Alexander RW, Schlant RC, Fuster V. New York, McGraw-Hill, 1998, pp 1833–1850.

20. Prosthetic Heart Valves

I **INTRODUCTION.** In the United States, more than 60,000 valve replacements are performed each year. Although more than 80 models of prosthetic heart valves have been developed, the models most commonly used are listed in Table 20-1.

II **PROSTHETIC VALVE TYPES**

A. **Bioprosthetic valves** are generally chosen for elderly patients who need aortic valve replacement and are poor candidates for anticoagulation therapy.

    1. **Structure.** Bioprosthetic valves may be **heterografts** or **homografts**.

        a. A **heterograft** valve is composed of a metal support that is covered with the valvular or pericardial tissue of a pig or cow (Figure 20-1).

        b. A **homograft** valve is a preserved human valve.

    2. **Durability.** Within 10–15 years of implantation, 30% of heterografts and 20% of homografts will fail. Patients younger than 40 years have a higher incidence of premature failure.

B. **Mechanical valves** are preferred for patients who need mitral or aortic valve replacement, are expected to live longer than 10–15 years, and are considered good candidates for anticoagulation therapy.

    1. **Structure.** Mechanical valves are composed of metal or carbon alloys, and are classified according to their structure:

        a. Caged-ball valves (e.g., Starr-Edwards valve)

        b. Single tilting-disk valves

        c. Bileaflet tilting-disk valves

    2. **Durability.** Mechanical valves are very durable, and almost always last at least 20–30 years.

III **APPROACH TO THE PATIENT**

A. Auscultation

    1. Normal findings

        a. **Bioprosthetic valves** produce heart sounds similar to those of native valves.

        b. **Mechanical valves** produce crisp, high-pitched opening and closing sounds. With a caged-ball valve, the opening sound is louder than the closing sound; the opposite occurs with a tilting-disk valve.

Table 20-1. Types of Prosthetic Heart Valves				
Type	Model	Durability	Thrombogenicity*	Recommended INR
Bioprosthetic				
Heterografts	Hancock porcine	Fair	++	2.0–3.0†
	Carpentier-Edwards	Fair	++	2.0–3.0†
	Ionescu-Shiley‡	Fair	+	2.0–3.0†
Homografts	—	Good	+	Not indicated
Mechanical				
Caged-ball valves	Starr-Edwards	Excellent	++++	4.0–4.9
Single tilting-disk valves	Bjork-Shiley‡	Excellent	+++	3.0–3.9
	Medtronic-Hall	Excellent	+++	3.0–3.9
Bileaflet tilting-disk valves	Carbomedics	Excellent	++	2.5–2.9
	Edwards-Duromedics‡	Excellent	++	2.5–2.9
	St. Jude	Excellent	++	2.5–2.9

INR = international normalized ratio.

*A single plus sign (+) denotes minimal thrombogenicity, while four plus signs denote maximal thrombogenicity.

†The recommended INR is only required for the first 3 months after implantation. Aspirin treatment is recommended longterm.

‡These models are no longer available in the United States.

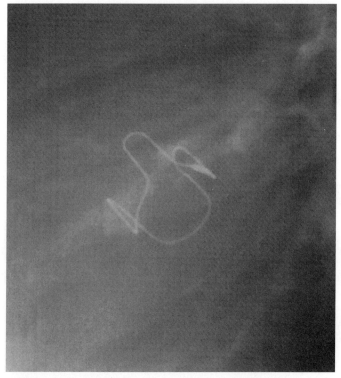

FIGURE 20-1. Magnified view of a lateral radiograph showing a Carpentier-Edwards porcine aortic valve. (Courtesy of C. Colangelo, M.D., San Francisco, CA)

2. Abnormal findings

a. Suspect valve dysfunction if there is a change in a preexisting murmur, an appearance of a new murmur, or a change in the intensity or quality of the opening or closing valve sounds.

b. A new flow murmur across a prosthetic valve may indicate valve thrombosis or pannus formation, both of which can lead to valvular stenosis.

HOT

KEY

Suspect endocarditis in any patient with a prosthetic valve who develops a fever.

B. Echocardiography

1. **Transthoracic echocardiography** (TTE) can be used to assess the structure and function of a prosthetic heart valve.

   a. **Two-dimensional echocardiography** (2DE) can be used to identify problems with bioprosthetic valves. This technique is not as useful with mechanical valves because of the echo reverberation caused by the metal.

   b. **Doppler echocardiography** is often helpful in diagnosing valve obstruction, and valvular or paravalvular regurgitation.

2. **Transesophageal echocardiography** (TEE) provides better resolution images of prosthetic heart valves compared with TTE, and is especially useful when endocarditis is suspected.

C. Cardiac catheterization. During cardiac catheterization, the pressure gradient across the prosthetic heart valve can be measured and the degree of regurgitation can be determined.

HOT   **KEY** Crossing a mechanical valve with a catheter should be avoided as it may cause severe acute valvular regurgitation.

D. Cinefluoroscopy is a useful, simple, and rapid technique that can be used to assess the structural integrity of mechanical valves. Valve obstruction (from thrombus or ingrown tissue), partial valve dehiscence (from excessive tilting or rocking of the ring), and valve fracture can be diagnosed.

HOT **KEY** Magnetic resonance imaging (MRI) can be safely performed in most patients with prosthetic heart valves after the immediate postoperative period. MRI should not be used in patients who received a Pre 6000 Starr-Edwards caged-ball valve from 1960–1964.

IV COMPLICATIONS

A. Prosthetic valve thrombosis

1. **Incidence.** Prosthetic valve thrombosis occurs in 0.1%–5.7% of patients per year. Valve thrombosis occurs at a similar rate in patients with bioprosthetic valves and those with adequate anticoagulation for mechanical valves.

2. **Risk factors** include

   a. Inadequate anticoagulation

   b. Prosthetic mitral valves

3. **Clinical presentation**
   a. Patients may present with pulmonary congestion, poor peripheral perfusion, and systemic embolization.
   b. The physical examination may reveal a new murmur, or a decrease in the intensity of the opening or closing valve sounds.
   c. Echocardiography or cinefluoroscopy may show decreased disk movement.
4. **Treatment**
   a. **Anticoagulation therapy.** Intravenous heparin should be started immediately. If the thrombus is smaller than 5 mm in diameter on echocardiography and is not obstructing the valve, anticoagulation therapy alone is sufficient treatment.
   b. **Thrombolytic therapy** [e.g., tissue plasminogen activator (t-PA)] is usually reserved for critically ill patients. Although it has a 70% success rate, it is also associated with a high risk of embolization (approximately 15%–20%).
   c. **Surgical therapy** may be required if valve obstruction is diagnosed. The perioperative mortality rate is approximately 15%.

B. **Embolization**
1. **Incidence**
   a. For patients with **bioprosthetic valves,** the incidence of major embolization (e.g., cerebrovascular event) is 1% per year.
   b. For patients with **mechanical valves,** the incidence of embolization is 4% per year without antithrombotic therapy, 2% per year with antiplatelet therapy, and 1% per year with warfarin.
2. **Risk factors** include
   a. Prosthetic mitral valves
   b. Multiple prosthetic valves
   c. Caged-ball valves
   d. Age greater than 70 years
   e. Atrial fibrillation
   f. A depressed left ventricular ejection fraction (LVEF)
3. **Clinical presentation**
   a. Patients usually present with a cerebrovascular accident.
   b. Diagnostic tests should be used to rule out prosthetic valve thrombosis and endocarditis.
4. **Treatment.** If a computed tomography (CT) scan shows no evidence of intracerebral bleeding and the patient's anticoagulant levels are subtherapeutic, heparin therapy should be restarted immediately.

C. **Structural failure**
1. **Incidence**
   a. **Bioprosthetic valves.** The incidence of structural failure is roughly 2%–3% of patients per year.

   b. Mechanical valves are very durable. The incidence of
      structural failure is no more than 0.5% of patients per
      year.
   2. Risk factors include
      a. Age less than 40 years
      b. Prosthetic mitral valves
   3. Clinical presentation
      a. Patients with **bioprosthetic valves** usually present with a
         gradual onset of dyspnea as a result of congestive heart
         failure (CHF) from valve regurgitation or stenosis.
      b. For patients with **mechanical valves,** strut failure can re-
         sult in the immediate onset of dyspnea, syncope, or car-
         diac arrest, all of which are caused by disk embolization
         and severe valve regurgitation.
   4. Treatment involves immediate valve replacement.
D. Hemolytic anemia may be caused by paravalvular leakage, partial dehiscence, or prosthetic valve endocarditis.
   1. Incidence. This is a rare complication in patients with pros-
      thetic heart valves.
   2. Risk factors include
      a. Multiple prosthetic valves
      b. Caged-ball valves
   3. Clinical presentation. Patients usually present with an in-
      creased cardiac output (CO) and tachycardia. Blood tests that
      reveal anemia, increased lactate dehydrogenase, decreased
      haptoglobin, and reticulocytosis can confirm the diagnosis.
   4. Treatment. Patients should receive iron and folate supple-
      ments, and blood transfusions. If the anemia remains refrac-
      tory to treatment, valve replacement may be performed.
E. Prosthetic valve endocarditis
   1. Incidence. Endocarditis occurs in 3%–6% of patients with a
      prosthetic heart valve, regardless of the type of valve used.
   2. Risk factor includes lack of appropriate antibiotic prophy-
      laxis (see Chapter 22).
   3. Clinical presentation
      a. Patients with prosthetic valve endocarditis usually present
         with an unexplained fever. Other manifestations include a
         new or changed murmur, systemic embolization, CHF, or a
         new conduction abnormality (e.g., a prolonged PR interval).
      b. Blood cultures can usually confirm the diagnosis. An ele-
         vated white blood cell count and erythrocyte sedimenta-
         tion rate (ESR) will usually be present.
      c. Echocardiography is useful for detecting vegetations and
         assessing regurgitation.
   4. Treatment
      a. Medical therapy. For patients with prosthetic valve strep-
         tococcal endocarditis, 50% can be cured with a 6- to 8-

week course of intravenous antibiotics. Blood cultures should be obtained once a week during treatment and continued for at least 1 month after completion of the antibiotic course. Interrupting anticoagulation therapy remains controversial.

b. Surgical therapy may be used for patients with prosthetic valve endocarditis and the following criteria:

(1) Positive blood cultures after 3–5 days of antibiotic therapy

(2) Reinfection after completion of the antibiotic course

(3) Major or recurrent embolization

(4) Ring abscess

(5) Valve obstruction

(6) Fungal infection in the prosthetic valve

V FOLLOW-UP

A. General measures

1. Patients should have an annual history and physical examination.

2. Prophylactic antibiotics should be administered to prevent infectious endocarditis (see Chapter 22).

B. Prevention of thromboembolism

1. Bioprosthetic valves

a. Patients with a heterograft valve should receive warfarin for the first 3 months after implantation to prevent thromboembolism. The target international normalized ratio (INR) is 2.0–3.0. Aspirin (325 mg/day) should then be used as long-term treatment.

b. Patients with a homograft valve do not need anticoagulation or antiplatelet therapy.

2. Mechanical valves. Because patients with mechanical valves are prone to developing blood clots, long-term anticoagulation therapy is required. The target INR depends on the type of mechanical valve used (see Table 20-1). Patients who have an increased risk for thromboembolism (see IV B 2) may require a higher target INR.

References

Grukemeier GL, Starr Albert, Rahimtoola SH: Clinical performance of prosthetic heart valves. In *Hurst's The Heart,* 9th ed. Edited by Alexander RW, Schlant RC, Fuster V. New York, McGraw-Hill, 1998, pp 1851–1866.

Vongpatanasin W, Hillis LD, Lange RA: Prosthetic heart valves. *N Engl J Med* 335(6):407–416, 1996.

PART VI

PERICARDIAL AND ENDOCARDIAL DISEASE

21. Pericardial Disease

I **INTRODUCTION.** Early diagnosis is important because pericardial disease often indicates another systemic illness that may be life threatening.

A. Anatomy
1. The **parietal pericardium** is the tough, fibrous outer layer of the pericardium, which attaches to the sternum and great vessels.
2. The **visceral pericardium** is the internal single-cell layer of the pericardium, which covers the surface of the heart.
3. The **pericardial cavity** (i.e., the space between the two layers of the pericardium) normally contains 15–50 mL of clear fluid.

B. Function. The function of the pericardium remains unclear because its congenital absence or surgical removal has no adverse consequences. The pericardium may shield the heart from inflammation and infection.

II **ACUTE PERICARDITIS** may be associated with a pericardial effusion (i.e., an exudation of fluid into the pericardial cavity).

A. Causes. Acute pericarditis may be **idiopathic,** or it may be caused by:
1. **Infection**
   a. **Viral infections** [e.g., Coxsackie B virus, echovirus, adenovirus, human immunodeficiency virus (HIV)]
   b. **Bacterial infections** (e.g., staphylococcal, streptococcal, pneumococcal, meningococcal infections, tuberculosis)
   c. **Fungal infections** (e.g., histoplasmosis, coccidioidomycosis, aspergillosis)
   d. **Protozoal infections** (e.g., amebiasis, toxoplasmosis)
2. **Malignancy** (primary and metastatic neoplasms)
3. **Connective tissue disorders** [e.g., systemic lupus erythematosus (SLE), rheumatoid arthritis, vasculitis]

4. **Dressler's syndrome** is a complication of myocardial infarction (MI) that may develop 1 week to several months after MI; it is thought to be due to an autoimmune process. Dressler's syndrome is characterized by pleuritic chest pain, fever, pericardial friction rub, and leukocytosis.
5. **Radiation therapy**
6. **Trauma** (e.g., pericardiotomy, blunt chest trauma, and iatrogenic injuries)
7. **Metabolic disorders** (e.g., uremia, myxedema)
8. **Medications** (e.g., hydralazine, procainamide, isoniazid, anticoagulants, methysergide)
9. **Congenital disorders** (e.g., pericardial cysts, thymic cysts)
10. **Other disorders** (e.g., aortic dissection, amyloidosis, sarcoidosis, familial Mediterranean fever)

B. **Approach to the patient**
 1. **Patient history**
   a. **Chest pain** typically presents as sharp discomfort in the retrosternal area that worsens when the patient lies down and improves when the patient sits up. The pain is usually "pleuritic," meaning it worsens during inspiration.

HOT ▶ **KEY** It is important to exclude other serious causes of chest pain [e.g., acute myocardial infarction (AMI), aortic dissection, pulmonary embolism, pneumothorax] before diagnosing the patient with acute pericarditis.

---

   b. **Dyspnea** may also be present.
   c. **Prodromal symptoms** include fever, myalgia, and malaise.
 2. **Physical examination**
   a. The **central venous pressure** (CVP) is normal in patients with uncomplicated acute pericarditis without a pericardial effusion.
   b. A **pericardial friction rub** is a scratchy sound commonly heard between the left lower sternal border and the cardiac apex. The rub is classically triphasic (with components in atrial systole, ventricular systole, and ventricular diastole), but it can also be biphasic or monophasic.
   c. **Distant heart sounds** may suggest a pericardial effusion.
 3. **Laboratory studies**
   a. Electrolytes, blood urea nitrogen (BUN), creatinine, a complete blood count (CBC), thyroid function tests, prothrombin time, and partial thromboplastin time should be ordered routinely.
   b. The erythrocyte sedimentation rate (ESR) is commonly elevated in patients with pericardial disease. This elevation, however, occurs in many different disorders.

   c. Cardiac enzymes should be drawn to exclude AMI or co-existing myocarditis.

   d. Blood cultures are indicated if bacterial pericarditis is suspected.

 4. Electrocardiography

   a. Early findings (within hours to days) include widespread ST-segment elevation, with depression of the PR segment below the baseline of the TP segment (Figure 21-1).

   b. Later findings (after several days to weeks) show a normal pattern followed by diffuse T-wave inversions.

HOT **KEY** Great care must be taken not to confuse acute pericarditis with AMI. The absence of Q waves and inverted T waves and the presence of upwardly concave ST segments support a diagnosis of acute pericarditis.

---

 5. Imaging studies

   a. Radiography. The chest radiograph is usually normal.

    (1) An enlarged cardiac silhouette may suggest a pericardial effusion (Figure 21- 2).

    (2) Mediastinal widening may indicate aortic dissection.

   b. Echocardiography. Pericardial effusion is detected in 60% of patients with pericarditis. It can also be used to help distinguish acute pericarditis from AMI.

C. Treatment. Treat the **underlying cause** of acute pericarditis first.

 1. Idiopathic or **viral infections**

   a. Aspirin (650 mg orally every 4 hours) or ibuprofen (800 mg orally every 8 hours) can be administered to relieve symptoms. Steroids are generally not effective.

   b. Anticoagulants (e.g., subcutaneous heparin) should be avoided because of the risk for intrapericardial hemorrhage.

 2. Bacterial infections that cause pericarditis are often treated as medical emergencies.

   a. Parenteral antibiotics should be immediately administered.

   b. Pericardiocentesis may be performed if pericardial effusion is present.

 3. Tuberculosis is associated with a high rate of pericardial effusion early in the course and constrictive pericarditis late in the course.

   a. Triple drug antituberculous therapy should be administered immediately (i.e., 300 mg isoniazid, 600 mg rifampin, and 25 mg/kg pyrazinamide daily).

   b. Pericardiocentesis may be performed if pericardial effusion is present.

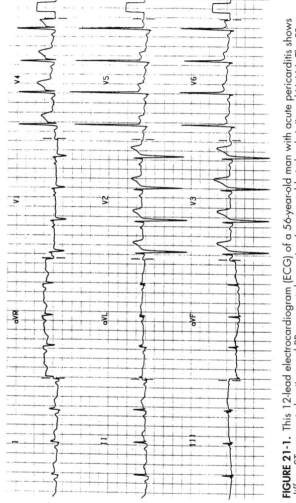

FIGURE 21-1. This 12-lead electrocardiogram (ECG) of a 56-year-old man with acute pericarditis shows diffuse ST-segment elevation and PR-segment depression (most notably in leads I, II, and V_4-V_6). The PR-segment elevation in lead aVR is referred to as the **"knuckle sign"** because it appears as if someone is pushing the segment up with a knuckle. (Courtesy of G. Thomas Evans Jr., M.D., University of California San Francisco, San Francisco, CA)

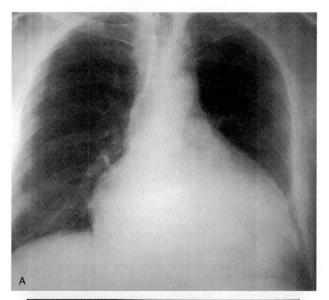

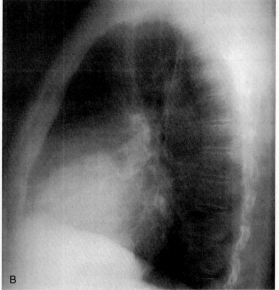

FIGURE 21-2. These (A) posteroanterior and (B) lateral chest films indicate cardiomegaly that is caused by a large pericardial effusion. The globular shape of the cardiac silhouette and the clear lung fields suggest pericardial effusion, as opposed to ventricular dysfunction, as the cause of cardiomegaly. (Courtesy of C. Colangelo, M.D., San Francisco, CA)

4. Malignancy

a. Chemotherapy may be used to treat the underlying malignancy. The diagnosis of malignant pericarditis often reflects widespread disease, which has a very poor prognosis.

b. Catheter or surgical drainage may be performed for recurrent pericardial effusions.

5. Dressler's syndrome

a. Nonsteroidal anti-inflammatory drugs (NSAIDs) may be administered to relieve symptoms.

b. Prednisone may be used for more resistant cases of pericarditis.

6. Uremia

a. Dialysis is the treatment of choice.

b. Catheter or surgical drainage may be performed for recurrent pericardial effusions.

III **CARDIAC TAMPONADE** occurs when a pericardial effusion is sufficiently large or rapid enough to impede ventricular filling (Figure 21-3A).

A. Causes. Trauma, cardiac rupture occurring during AMI, and aortic dissection are the most common causes of acute cardiac tamponade.

HOT

KEY
Iatrogenic injuries causing cardiac perforation can occur during cardiac catheterization or pacemaker implantation.

B. Approach to the patient. Cardiac tamponade is a clinical diagnosis based on specific symptoms and signs.

1. Patient history. Dyspnea and lightheadedness may indicate cardiac tamponade.

2. Physical examination

a. CVP

(1) An elevation in the pericardial pressure will cause an elevation in the CVP, leading to jugular venous distention.

(2) Tachycardia and hypotension may indicate cardiac tamponade.

b. Chest examination reveals clear lung fields.

HOT

KEY
Pulmonary edema is usually absent in patients with cardiac tamponade.

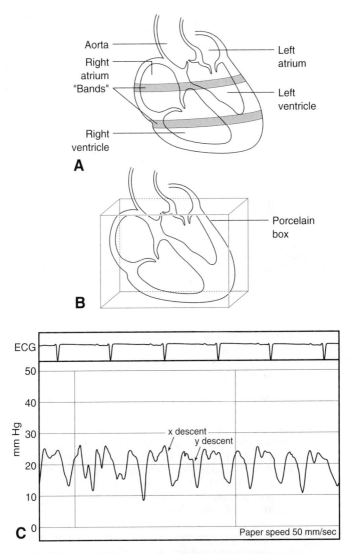

FIGURE 21-3. (*A*) **Cardiac tamponade** can be likened to a heart being squeezed by rubber bands. Ventricular filling is restricted throughout the entire cardiac cycle. Right atrial pressure is increased and the *y* descent is absent. (*B*) **Constrictive pericarditis** can be likened to a heart being constrained within a porcelain box. Early ventricular filling is rapid; however, when the ventricles fill to the limits of the box, ventricular filling slows and the filling pressures abruptly rise. (*C*) Right atrial pressure tracings show prominent *x* and *y* descents in **constrictive pericarditis.** (*continued*)

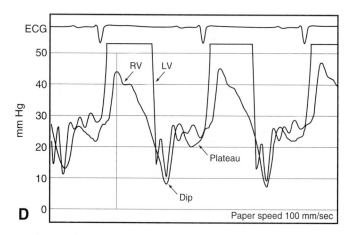

D

FIGURE 21-3. (*CONTINUED*) (*D*) The classic dip-and-plateau pattern seen in **constrictive pericarditis** results from the rapid ventricular filling in early diastole (dip) which corresponds to the prominant *y* descent in the right atrial pressure tracing. The abrupt rise in filling pressures reflects slow ventricular filling throughout the remainder of diastole (plateau).

    c. Pulsus paradoxus (i.e., a decrease in the systolic blood pressure by more than 10 mm Hg during inspiration) is usually present in patients with cardiac tamponade. Pulsus paradoxus can be measured using the following steps:
       (1) Manually inflate the blood pressure cuff above the systolic pressure and then slowly release it.
       (2) Initially, the blood pressure sounds (i.e., Korotkoff sounds) are heard only during expiration. As the cuff pressure is reduced, the sounds are heard continuously.
       (3) Pulse paradoxus is calculated as the difference in pressure when the Korotkoff sounds are heard only during expiration and the pressure when the sounds are heard continuously.

HOT

KEY

Pulsus paradoxus results from increased filling of the right heart chambers during inspiration. The increased venous return to the right side of the heart causes the interventricular septum to bulge into the left ventricle, leading to decreased filling of the left ventricle. The subsequent decrease in stroke volume accounts for the drop in blood pressure during inspiration.

3. Electrocardiography
   a. Sinus tachycardia with low QRS voltage may be present.
   b. Electrical alternans is diagnosed when the height of the QRS varies from complex to complex. This results from shifting of the axis as the heart rocks back and forth in the pericardial effusion.
4. Echocardiography. This is the most useful diagnostic test and should be immediately performed in patients with suspected tamponade (Figure 21-4). If the pericardial effusion is large enough to result in **cardiac tamponade,** the echocardiogram may show:
   a. A diastolic collapse of the right atrium and ventricle
   b. Respiratory variation in the tricuspid and mitral inflow velocities
   c. A dilated inferior vena cava

C. Treatment. For patients with cardiac tamponade, the only effective treatment is drainage. There are three options for removing pericardial fluid.
   1. Diagnostic **pericardiocentesis,** therapeutic pericardiocentesis, or both can be performed at the bedside or in the cardiac catheterization laboratory. A catheter can be left in place for several days for large or recurrent effusions.

HOT KEY

Intravascular volume expansion and dopamine may be helpful while preparing a hypotensive patient with tamponade for pericardiocentesis.

---

2. Balloon pericardiotomy may be performed in the cardiac catheterization laboratory in selected patients with recurrent pericardial effusions.
3. Surgical drainage of the pericardium may be performed using the subxiphoid approach while the patient is under local anesthesia.

IV CONSTRICTIVE PERICARDITIS is a late complication of pericarditis (see Figure 21-3B).

A. Approach to the patient
   1. Patient history. Constrictive pericarditis usually has a slow, insidious onset. Symptoms are usually nonspecific and include dyspnea, fatigue, a growing abdominal girth, and lower extremity edema.
   2. Physical examination
      a. The **CVP** will be elevated with prominent x and y descents (see Figure 21-3C).

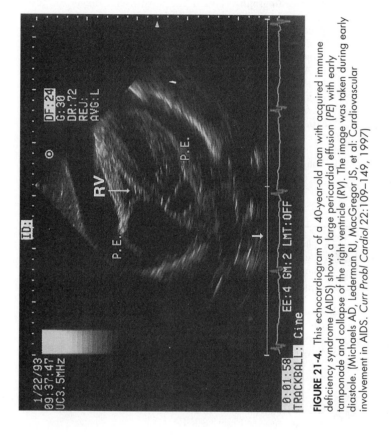

FIGURE 21-4. This echocardiogram of a 40-year-old man with acquired immune deficiency syndrome (AIDS) shows a large pericardial effusion (*PE*) with early tamponade and collapse of the right ventricle (*RV*). The image was taken during early diastole. (Michaels AD, Lederman RJ, MacGregor JS, et al: Cardiovascular involvement in AIDS. *Curr Probl Cardiol* 22:109–149, 1997)

    b. Kussmaul's sign (i.e., an increase in the CVP during inspiration) is usually present in patients with constrictive pericarditis.

3. Imaging studies

    a. Echocardiography. Constrictive pericarditis can be suggested with specific echocardiographic findings, which include:

        (1) The absence of normal "sliding" between the pericardial layers (suggesting pericardial adhesions)

        (2) Pericardial thickening

    b. Radiography. A calcified pericardium raises the possibility of constrictive pericarditis.

    c. Magnetic resonance imaging (MRI) of the heart may be useful in measuring pericardial thickening.

    d. Cardiac catheterization can help confirm the diagnosis of constrictive pericarditis.

        (1) Diastolic pressure equalization between both atria and ventricles may be demonstrated. Recordings from the right and left ventricles show elevated diastolic pressures with the classic dip-and-plateau pattern (see Figure 21-3D).

        (2) The right atrial pressure shows prominent x and y descents (see Figure 21-3C).

B. Treatment

    1. Symptoms should be relieved using medical therapy. For example, in patients with clinical evidence of volume overload, sodium restriction and diuretics (e.g., furosemide) may be helpful.

    2. Surgical pericardiectomy (i.e., pericardial stripping) should be performed in patients with severe symptoms. It may take several weeks to months for the cardiac-filling pattern to normalize after pericardial stripping. The risk of perioperative mortality is approximately 5%-15%.

References

Osterberg L, Vagelos R, Atwood JE: Case presentation and review: constrictive pericarditis. *West J Med* 169(4):232–239, 1998.

Shabetai R: Disease of the pericardium. In *Hurst's The Heart,* 9th ed. Edited by Alexander RW, Schlant RC, Fuster V. New York, McGraw-Hill, 1998, pp 2169–2204.

22. Endocarditis

I INTRODUCTION

A. Appropriately diagnosing and treating infective endocarditis usually leads to a good outcome, whereas failure to deliver proper therapy often results in serious morbidity and mortality.

B. Typically, **acute endocarditis** results from *Staphylococcus aureus* infection of previously normal valves and may result in rapid valvular dysfunction and death. **Subacute endocarditis** is usually caused by *Streptococcus viridans* infection of previously abnormal valves and has a slower course. Overlap between these two presentations does occur.

C. Prevention of endocarditis with antibiotic prophylaxis is important in high-risk patients undergoing certain medical procedures (see VIII).

II CAUSES OF ENDOCARDITIS

A. *Streptococcus viridans* (*Streptococcus salivarius, Streptococcus sanguis, Streptococcus mitior, and Streptococcus milleri*), **enterococci,** and *Streptococcus bovis* (nonenterococcal group D streptococci) account for most cases of native valve endocarditis in patients without a history of intravenous drug use (IVDU).

   1. Approximately 15%–20% of endocarditis caused by *S viridans* develops after a dental procedure.

   2. Approximately 50% of endocarditis caused by an enterococcal infection develops after a genitourinary or gastrointestinal procedure.

B. *Staphylococcus aureus* and *Staphylococcus epidermidis* are the most common causes of IVDU-related endocarditis and prosthetic valve endocarditis, respectively.

C. **Gram-negative bacteria** can cause endocarditis, usually in association with genitourinary or gastrointestinal procedures or surgery.

D. **Culture-negative organisms** may cause endocarditis in patients who have recently received antibiotics or who have been infected with certain microorganisms.

   1. HACEK group organisms. *Haemophilus parainfluenzae/ Haemophilus aphrophilus, Actinobacillus actinomycetemcomitans, Cardiobacterium hominis, Eikenella corrodens,* and *Kingella kingae* are Gram-negative bacilli that grow slowly and account for 5%–10% of native valve endocarditis in patients without a history of IVDU. Ask the microbiology laboratory to save the blood cultures for a prolonged period (i.e., at least 2 weeks) if culture-negative endocarditis is suspected.

2. **Fungi.** Large vegetations are often found in patients with endocarditis associated with *Candida* or *Aspergillus* infection. Susceptible patients usually are immunocompromised. An intravascular source is frequently noted (e.g., an indwelling intravenous catheter). Specific fungal cultures may be required.

3. **Rickettsia** (*Coxiella burnetii*) and **chlamydia** (*Chlamydia psittaci* and *Chlamydia trachomatis*) are rare causes of culture-negative endocarditis.

III CLINICAL MANIFESTATIONS OF ENDOCARDITIS. The clinical manifestations of endocarditis vary, but most closely depend on which organism is involved and whether the patient has left-sided (aortic or mitral) or right-sided (usually tricuspid) disease (Figure 22-1).

A. **Fever** occurs in almost all patients; however, elderly patients and patients taking steroids or nonsteroidal anti-inflammatory drugs (NSAIDs) may be afebrile.

B. **Murmurs** are almost always present. Because murmurs are often not prominent, however, their significance may be underestimated.

C. **Low back pain, arthralgias,** and **myalgias** are very common.

D. **Splenomegaly** may occur with subacute endocarditis.

E. **Classic findings,** including **Osler's nodes, Janeway lesions, Roth spots** (retinal hemorrhages), **petechiae of the palate or conjunctiva,** and **splinter hemorrhages** (beneath the nailbed) are rarely found.

HOT KEY — Although Osler's nodes are typically violaceous lesions located on the tips of the fingers or toes, and Janeway lesions are typically erythematous patches located on the palms or soles, the predominant distinction between the two is that **Osler's nodes** are **painful** whereas **Janeway lesions** are **painless.**

IV COMPLICATIONS OF ENDOCARDITIS

A. **Congestive heart failure (CHF).** Pulmonary edema and hypotension may occur with significant left-sided (aortic or mitral) valve regurgitation, whereas peripheral edema may result from right-sided (tricuspid) regurgitation.

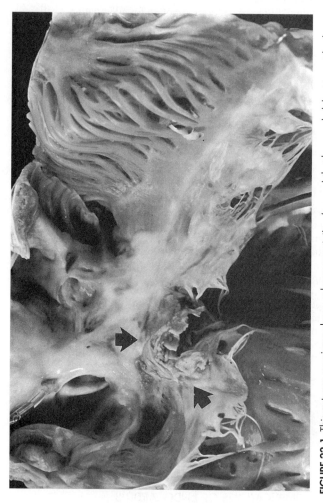

FIGURE 22-1. This autopsy specimen shows a large vegetation (*arrows*) that has eroded the tricuspid valve. The subsequent perforation at the commissure between the septal and anterosuperior leaflets caused severe tricuspid insufficiency. (Courtesy of P.C. Ursell, M.D., San Francisco, CA)

B. Myocardial abscess formation may lead to bradycardia with varying degrees of atrioventricular (AV) block.

C. Septic emboli. Left-sided endocarditis may result in a peripheral infarct (e.g., cerebrovascular accident, meningitis, brain abscess, renal infarction), whereas right-sided endocarditis may cause septic emboli with pulmonary infarction, pulmonary abscess, or both.

D. Purulent pericarditis is a rare complication that requires surgical drainage.

V APPROACH TO THE PATIENT

A. Patient history

1. Endocarditis is a diagnosis that is often missed. Therefore, it should be suspected in patients with chronic fatigue, fever of unknown origin, and nonspecific arthralgias and myalgias.

2. Be sure to ask the patient about risk factors for endocarditis (i.e., known valvular disease, recent procedures or surgery, IVDU).

B. Physical examination. In addition to performing a complete physical examination, pay special attention to the:

1. **Cardiac examination** (to detect pathologic murmurs)

2. **Fundoscopic examination** (to search for Roth spots)

3. **Skin examination** (to search for Osler's nodes, Janeway lesions, and petechiae)

HOT **KEY** Patients who have an unexplained fever and a low clinical probability of endocarditis, are conscientious about follow-up, and appear well can sometimes be evaluated as outpatients. Active intravenous drug users with a fever and no obvious alternative source of infection are almost always admitted to rule out endocarditis.

C. Diagnostic tests

1. **Blood cultures** are the **gold standard** for diagnosis. Two to three sets of aerobic and anaerobic cultures are usually obtained.

   a. Different venous sites are usually used to avoid confounding skin contamination. The femoral venous site should be avoided.

   b. Cultures should be taken before initiating antibiotic therapy.

2. **Erythrocyte sedimentation rate (ESR).** Although a low ESR (i.e., ≤ 20 mm/hr) decreases the likelihood of endocarditis, an elevated ESR does not confirm the diagnosis.

3. **Urinalysis.** The presence of *S. aureus* in the urine is highly suggestive of endocarditis.

4. Electrocardiography. Endocarditis with AV block often indicates a valvular ring abscess.

5. Chest radiography. Pulmonary cavities may indicate septic emboli from a tricuspid valve vegetation.

6. Echocardiography. Because the prognosis and the duration of therapy may differ depending on which side of the heart is involved, echocardiography is often performed to define which valve is infected.

  a. Transthoracic echocardiography (TTE) is often performed first and can detect vegetations in approximately 60% of patients with endocarditis.

  b. Transesophageal echocardiography (TEE) can detect vegetations in approximately 95% of patients with endocarditis. TEE can also determine more accurately the size and location of the vegetations.

D. Prognosis. Patients with the following clinical characteristics have a less favorable prognosis:

  1. Advanced age
  2. CHF
  3. Endocarditis associated with a fungal infection
  4. Aortic valve involvement
  5. Prosthetic valve involvement
  6. A valvular ring abscess
  7. A large vegetation

VI TREATMENT

A. Empiric therapy

  1. Suspected acute endocarditis is a common consideration in intravenous drug users with a fever. *S. aureus* can destroy the valve (usually tricuspid) quickly, so therapy is initiated immediately after blood cultures are drawn.

    a. Nafcillin plus gentamicin is often used in regions where the incidence of methicillin-resistant *S. aureus* (MRSA) is low. **Ampicillin** is occasionally added to this regimen if enterococcal infection is suspected.

    b. Vancomycin plus gentamicin may be administered in regions where the incidence of MRSA is high.

  2. Suspected subacute endocarditis may be treated with penicillin and an aminoglycoside. Because the consequences of not treating *S. aureus* infection can be severe, this regimen should only be considered in patients with a chronic and very stable course.

  3. Suspected prosthetic valve endocarditis may be treated with vancomycin and an aminoglycoside. This regimen will cover methicillin-resistant *S. epidermidis* while treating possible enterococcal infection as well.

B. Organism-specific therapy. The duration of therapy varies depending on whether the disease is right- or left-sided and on the minimal inhibitory concentration (MIC) of the antibacterial needed to inhibit organism growth.

1. *S viridans* **infections** are usually treated with penicillin and an aminoglycoside (Table 22-1).

2. **Enterococcal infections** usually require prolonged treatment with 4–6 weeks of penicillin G plus gentamicin. Depending on the MIC, ampicillin or vancomycin may need to be substituted for penicillin.

3. **Staphylococcal infections**
   a. **Methicillin-sensitive** *S aureus* **(MSSA) infections** may be treated with at least 6 weeks of nafcillin (2 g intravenously every 4 hours) plus 2 weeks of gentamicin (1 mg/kg intravenously every 8 hours).
      (1) For complicated cases and those involving prosthetic valves, rifampin (300 mg orally every 8 hours) may be added.
      (2) For uncomplicated, right-sided endocarditis caused by IVDU, 2 weeks of nafcillin plus gentamicin is effective.
   b. **MRSA infections** may be treated with at least 6 weeks of vancomycin (1 g intravenously every 12 hours) and rifampin, plus 2 weeks of gentamicin.

TABLE 22-1. Treatment for Patients with *Streptococcal viridans* Infection

Sensitivity to Penicillin	Minimal Inhibitory Concentration	Treatment*
Penicillin- susceptible strains	≤0.1 µg/mL	4 weeks of penicillin G (12–18 million units daily), or 2 weeks of penicillin G plus gentamicin†
Relatively penicillin-resistant strains	> 0.1 µg/mL and < 0.5 µg/mL	4 weeks of penicillin G (18 million units daily) plus 2 weeks of gentamicin†
Penicillin-resistant strains	≥0.5 µg/mL	4–6 weeks of penicillin G (18–30 million units daily) plus gentamicin†

*All drugs should be administered intravenously.
†The dose of gentamicin is 1 mg/kg every 8 hours.

4. **HACEK group infections** can be treated with 4 weeks of ceftriaxone (2 g intravenously daily). Alternatively, patients can be treated with 4 weeks of ampicillin plus gentamicin.

C. **Surgery.** Valve replacement is often indicated when:

1. Fungal infection is present.
2. A prosthetic valve is infected.
3. Complications (e.g., myocardial abscess, acute valvular regurgitation with CHF) have developed.
4. Medical therapy has failed, with persistent bacteremia for 10 days or longer.
5. The patient has experienced more than one embolic event.

VII FOLLOW-UP

A. **Frequent examinations** are essential. Listen carefully for a new or changing murmur, look for embolic phenomena, and watch for widening of the pulse pressure (which would suggest possible aortic regurgitation).

1. **Bilateral disease.** Although intravenous drug users more commonly have right-sided disease, they may also have left-sided or bilateral endocarditis.
2. **Persistent fever.** Defervescence usually occurs within 1 week, but prolonged fevers may be noted with *S aureus* infection. Drug reactions are a common cause of persistent or recurrent fever, but myocardial or metastatic abscess formation should always be considered (especially with *S aureus* infection).

B. **Electrocardiograms (ECGs).** An ECG should be obtained on admission and daily during hospitalization. Prolongation of the PR interval should prompt an echocardiogram to evaluate possible myocardial abscess formation.

VIII RISK STRATIFICATION

A. **Risk assessment**

1. An **underlying cardiac abnormality** may increase a patient's risk of developing endocarditis (Table 22-2). Approximately 60%–80% of patients with native valve endocarditis have an underlying cardiac abnormality.
   a. **High-risk patients** should receive antibiotic prophylaxis before certain medical procedures.
   b. **Intermediate-risk patients** potentially may benefit from antibiotic prophylaxis.
   c. **Low-risk patients** are generally not considered candidates for antibiotic prophylaxis.
2. **Certain medical procedures** may also increase a patient's risk of developing endocarditis. Prophylaxis is usually re-

TABLE 22-2. Risk of Endocarditis Associated With an Underlying Cardiac Abnormality	
Patient Risk	**Underlying Cardiac Abnormality**
High	Prosthetic heart valves Previous endocarditis Aortic or mitral stenosis or regurgitation Arteriovenous fistula Marfan's syndrome Particular types of congenital heart disease (e.g., PDA, VSD, tetralogy of Fallot, aortic coarctation)
Intermediate	MVP with regurgitation Tricuspid or pulmonary valve disease Hypertrophic cardiomyopathy
Low	MVP without regurgitation Isolated ASD Cardiac pacemaker Previous bypass surgery or angioplasty

ASD = atrial septal defect; MVP = mitral valve prolapse; PDA = patent ductus arteriosus; VSD = ventricular septal defect.

quired for intermediate- or high-risk patients undergoing a high-risk procedure.

a. High-risk procedures include:

    (1) Dental procedures that are likely to cause bleeding (e.g., cleaning, extraction, and oral surgery)

    (2) Tonsillectomy, adenoidectomy, and rigid bronchoscopy

    (3) Sclerotherapy for esophageal varices, esophageal stricture dilatation, and gallbladder surgery

    (4) Abortion, urethral dilatation, urethral catheterization in a patient with infection, cytoscopy, and prostatectomy

b. Low-risk procedures include:

    (1) Simple fillings above the gum line

    (2) Cardiac catheterization and TEE

    (3) Flexible bronchoscopy (with or without biopsy) and endotracheal intubation

    (4) Endoscopy (with or without biopsy), barium enema, and liver biopsy

    (5) Caesarean section, insertion of an intrauterine device, and urethral catheterization in a patient without infection

TABLE 22-3. Antibiotic Regimen for Patients Undergoing a Dental, Esophageal, or Upper Respiratory Procedure

Patient Risk	Sensitivity to Penicillin	Oral Administration*	Parenteral Administration†
Intermediate- and high-risk patients	Not allergic to penicillin	Amoxicillin (2 g)	Ampicillin (2 g)
	Allergic to penicillin	Clindamycin (600 mg), cephalexin (2 g), azithromycin (500 mg), or clarithromycin (500 mg)	Clindamycin (600 mg) or cefazolin (1 g)

*The oral dose should be administered 1 hour before the procedure.
†The intravenous or intramuscular dose should be administered 30 minutes before the procedure.
†Although oral administration is adequate, parenteral administration may also be used. The intravenous or intramuscular dose should be administered 30 minutes before the procedure.

TABLE 22-4. Antibiotic Regimen for Patients Undergoing a Gastrointestinal (Excluding Esophageal) or Genitourinary Procedure

Patient Risk	Sensitivity to Penicillin	Oral Administration*	Parenteral Administration†
Intermediate	Not allergic to penicillin	Amoxicillin (2 g)	Ampicillin (2 g)
	Allergic to penicillin	—	Vancomycin (1 g)
High	Not allergic to penicillin	—	Ampicillin (2 g) plus gentamicin (1.5 mg/kg)‡
	Allergic to penicillin	—	Vancomycin (1 g) plus gentamicin (1.5 mg/kg)

*The oral dose should be administered 1 hour before the procedure.
†The intravenous or intramuscular dose should be administered 30 minutes before the procedure.
‡Administer ampicillin (1 g intravenously or intramuscularly) or amoxicillin (1 g orally) 6 hours later.

B. Antibiotic prophylaxis regimens may reduce a patient's risk of developing endocarditis. Tables 22-3 and 22-4 provide the appropriate antibiotic regimens based on the patient's risk and the procedure being performed.

References

Dajani AS, Taubert KA, Wilson W, et al: Prevention of bacterial endocarditis. Recommendations by the American Heart Association. *Circulation* 96(1):358–366, 1997.

Durak DT: Infective endocarditis. In *Hurst's The Heart,* 9th ed. Edited by Alexander RW, Schlant RC, Fuster V. New York, McGraw- Hill, 1998, pp 2205–2239.

Wilson WR, Karchmer AW, Dajani AS, et al: Antibiotic treatment of adults with infective endocarditis due to streptococci, enterococci, staphylococci, and HACEK microorganisms. American Heart Association *JAMA* 274(21):1706–1713, 1995.

PART VII

HYPERTENSION

23. Systemic Hypertension

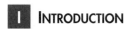 INTRODUCTION

A. Definitions

1. **Hypertension.** Over 50 million Americans have hypertension, which is defined as a systolic blood pressure of 140 mm Hg or greater or a diastolic blood pressure of 90 mm Hg or greater.

2. A **hypertensive urgency** is defined as Stage 4 hypertension (Table 23-1) but no end-organ damage.

3. A **hypertensive emergency** (e.g., malignant hypertension) is defined as an acute condition with Stage 4 hypertension (see Table 23-1) and end-organ damage [e.g., hypertensive encephalopathy, intracranial hemorrhage, acute myocardial infarction (AMI) or unstable angina, aortic dissection, eclampsia].

HOT KEY

A hypertensive emergency will develop in 1%–2% of patients with hypertension.

B. Untreated hypertension is associated with increased overall mortality and morbidity because of cardiac and renal damage. Although treatment improves the patient's prognosis, only 75% of those with hypertension are aware of their condition, only 50% of diagnosed patients are receiving medications, and less than 30% of treated patients have a blood pressure lower than 140/90 mm Hg.

II CAUSES OF HYPERTENSION

A. Primary (essential) hypertension has no identifiable cause and accounts for more than 90% of all cases of hypertension.

B. Secondary hypertension has an identifiable cause and accounts for 5%–10% of all cases. Causes include:

TABLE 23-1. Blood Pressure Classification for Adults			
	Blood Pressure (mm Hg)		
Category	Systolic		Diastolic
Optimal	< 120	and	< 80
Normal	< 130	and	< 85
High-normal	130–139	or	85–89
Hypertension			
Stage 1	140–159	or	90–99
Stage 2	160–179	or	100–109
Stage 3	180–209	or	110–119
Stage 4	≥ 210	or	≥ 120

1. **Renal arterial diseases.** Renovascular hypertension usually results from atherosclerosis or fibrous dysplasia. Renal artery stenosis is the most common curable cause of secondary hypertension but accounts for fewer than 3% of cases.

2. **Renal parenchymal diseases.** Reversible hypertension can occur in patients with acute renal disease. Irreversible hypertension can occur in patients with chronic end-stage renal disease.

3. **Endocrine disorders**

   a. **Primary hyperaldosteronism** (i.e., a syndrome associated with excess secretion of the adrenal mineralocorticoid aldosterone) is caused by either an aldosterone-producing adrenal adenoma (e.g., Conn's syndrome) or bilateral adrenal hyperplasia.

   b. **Cushing's syndrome** results from increased production of cortisol by the adrenal gland. Bilateral adrenal hyperplasia or adrenocorticotropic hormone (ACTH)-secreting pituitary tumors are the most common causes.

   c. **Pheochromocytomas** are tumors that produce catecholamines. Ninety percent of these tumors are located in the adrenal glands.

   d. **Hypothyroidism, hyperthyroidism,** and **hyperparathyroidism** are rare endocrine causes of secondary hypertension.

4. **Coarctation of the aorta** is a congenital anomaly located below the origin of the left subclavian artery in more than 95% of adult cases. Making this diagnosis is particularly important because more than 80% of these patients who do not receive corrective surgery will eventually die prematurely from complications of hypertension.

5. **Substance abuse** (e.g., excessive alcohol, cocaine)
6. **Medications** [e.g., cold preparations such as phenyl-propanolamine, monoamine oxidase (MAO) inhibitors, steroids, cyclosporine, oral contraceptives]

III CONSEQUENCES OF LONG-STANDING HYPERTENSION

A. **Cardiac complications.** Elevated blood pressure increases the risk of developing a variety of cardiac disorders.
   1. **Myocardial ischemia and infarction.** Hypertension can lead to progressive coronary atherosclerosis and left ventricular hypertrophy (LVH). These conditions may contribute to decreased myocardial oxygen supply and increased demand, respectively.
   2. **Congestive heart failure (CHF).** Hypertension can eventually lead to left ventricular dilatation with or without systolic and diastolic dysfunction.
B. **Vascular complications**
   1. **Stroke.** Hemorrhagic and thrombotic strokes are strongly associated with elevated blood pressure.
   2. **Aortic dissection and aneurysm formation** of the thoracic and abdominal aorta are complications of long-standing, severe hypertension.
   3. **Peripheral vascular disease,** leading to claudication and impotence, represents another complication of hypertension.
C. **Hypertensive retinopathy** can range from retinal arteriole constriction, sclerosis, and arteriovenous nicking to more severe manifestations such as hemorrhages, exudates, and papilledema.
D. **Hypertensive nephropathy**
   1. **Microalbuminuria** is an early abnormality of hypertensive renal disease.
   2. **Renal failure** with elevated serum blood urea nitrogen (BUN) and creatinine can develop with long-standing, severe hypertension.

IV HYPERTENSIVE EMERGENCY AND HYPERTENSIVE URGENCY

A. **Approach to the patient**
   1. **Patient history.** The following symptoms may signify a hypertensive emergency, necessitating an expedited work-up and early initiation of therapy:
      a. **Chest pain** caused by myocardial ischemia, MI, or aortic dissection

    b. Headache, confusion, or **altered mental status** caused by hypertensive encephalopathy or stroke

    c. Blurred vision from papilledema

    d. Hematuria from acute renal dysfunction

  2. Physical examination

    a. Vital signs. Patients with a systolic blood pressure of 210 mm Hg or greater or a diastolic blood pressure of 120 mm Hg or greater should have an expedited evaluation to rule out hypertensive emergency.

    b. Fundoscopic examination. With the patient's pupils dilated, assess for hemorrhage and papilledema.

    c. Cardiac examination. Evaluate the heart for evidence of left ventricular enlargement (e.g., diffuse and displaced apical impulse) and systolic dysfunction [e.g., a third heart sound (S_3)].

    d. Neurologic examination. Perform a screening mental status examination. Assess the patient for new focal neurologic deficits that could result from hypertensive encephalopathy or stroke.

  3. Laboratory studies

    a. The renal panel, including serum electrolytes, BUN, and creatinine, is important in the work-up of a patient with suspected hypertensive emergency.

    b. Test the urine for hematuria.

  4. Electrocardiography. Evidence of myocardial ischemia or infarction places the patient at an increased risk for complications and thus dictates a more aggressive approach to antihypertensive therapy.

B. Treatment

  1. Unstable patients with hypertensive emergency. Aggressive and rapid control of hypertension is paramount.

    a. Treatment goal. The immediate goal is to reduce the blood pressure by roughly 25% within the first 2 hours, then to approximately 160/100 mm Hg within 2–6 hours.

> **HOT KEY**
> Lowering the arterial blood pressure to "normal" levels in a patient having a hypertensive crisis may precipitate cerebral, cardiac, or renal ischemia. In general, sublingual or short-acting oral antihypertensive agents (particularly nifedipine) should be avoided because of the possibility of an excessive hypotensive response.

    b. Pharmacologic therapy involves administering antihypertensive drugs intravenously, and closely monitoring the hemodynamics in a coronary care unit (CCU).

   (1) Nitroprusside (0.3–10 µg/kg/min intravenous infusion) is generally the drug of choice for a hypertensive emergency. This vasodilator may be the most effective antihypertensive drug and can be titrated to effect. Adverse effects include nausea, cyanide and thiocyanate intoxication (after 2 days of therapy), and methemoglobinemia.

   (2) Labetalol (20–80 mg intravenous bolus every 10 minutes) has β-blocking and α-adrenergic-blocking activity. It is often used for patients with tachycardia, aortic dissection, or myocardial ischemia. Adverse effects include bronchospasm, heart block, and left ventricular systolic dysfunction.

   (3) Nitroglycerin (10–200 µg/min intravenous infusion) is often used for patients with suspected myocardial ischemia or infarction. Adverse effects include headache, tachycardia, and methemoglobinemia.

2. Stable patients with hypertensive urgency

  a. Treatment goal. The treatment of a patient with hypertensive urgency can take place over 12–24 hours. Hospitalization may not be required if oral antihypertensive therapy can be started and close follow-up ensured.

  b. Pharmacologic therapy

   (1) Oral antihypertensive agents (e.g., clonidine 0.1 mg or captopril 25 mg) can often be used to treat hypertensive urgency. If the patient is asymptomatic and blood pressure has improved (i.e., a systolic blood pressure less than 180 mm Hg and a diastolic blood pressure less than 110 mm Hg) following therapy, the patient could be sent home for follow-up the next day.

   (2) Intravenous antihypertensive agents may be considered for hospitalized patients.

V CHRONIC HYPERTENSION

A. Approach to the patient. The goal of the work-up is twofold: to determine the cause of the hypertension (i.e., primary or secondary) and to assess the patient for evidence of end-organ damage.

  1. Preliminary evaluation

   a. Patient history

    (1) Symptoms

     (a) Weight loss or gain, sweating, myalgias, flushing, or **palpitations** may signify an endocrine disorder causing secondary hypertension.

     (b) Fatigue and **pruritus** may be symptoms of renal failure, either as a complication of essential hypertension or as a cause of secondary hypertension.

   (c) **Dyspnea, orthopnea,** or **pedal edema** may be symptoms of CHF.

   (d) **Claudication, transient ischemic attacks,** or **impotence** may indicate peripheral vascular disease occurring as a complication of hypertension.

  (2) **Diet and drug history**

   (a) **Dietary salt and potassium intake**

   (b) **Medication use** (e.g., antihypertensive drugs, cold remedies, diet pills, MAO inhibitors, cyclosporine, oral contraceptives, steroids, and tricyclic antidepressants)

   (c) **Substance abuse** (e.g., tobacco, alcohol, and cocaine)

  (3) **Family history.** Determine if there is a family history of coronary heart disease, hypertension, or an inheritable secondary cause of hypertension (e.g., renal disease, hyperparathyroidism, pheochromocytoma, renovascular hypertension, thyroid disorder).

 b. Physical examination

  (1) **Vital signs.** In the stable patient, measure the blood pressure and heart rate carefully using the appropriate cuff size in both arms with the patient seated after at least 5 minutes of rest. Two or more readings at least 2 minutes apart are recommended.

HOT KEY

In the patient with coarctation of the aorta, the blood pressure in the arms is usually higher than that in the legs.

---

  (2) **Head and neck examination**

   (a) **Fundoscopic examination.** After the patient's pupils are dilated, assess for arteriovenous nicking, hemorrhage, and exudate.

   (b) **Neck examination.** Examine the neck for carotid bruits, jugular venous distention, and thyroid gland enlargement or masses.

  (3) **Cardiac examination.** A fourth heart sound (S_4) is frequently encountered in patients with LVH. A murmur of aortic regurgitation can suggest aortic root dilatation caused by long-standing hypertension.

  (4) **Abdominal examination**

   (a) **Abdominal bruits** may suggest renovascular disease, particularly if the bruits are unilateral and continue into diastole.

       (b) Palpable kidneys are often present in patients with polycystic kidney disease.

    (5) Extremity examination. Evaluate the extremities for peripheral edema and peripheral bruits. Diminished peripheral pulses in the lower extremities could represent peripheral vascular disease or, much less commonly, coarctation of the aorta.

    (6) Neurologic examination. Assess for focal neurologic deficits, which can be a complication of hypertension, and muscle weakness, which is seen in hyperaldosteronism and Cushing's syndrome.

  c. Laboratory studies

    (1) Complete blood count (CBC)

    (2) Renal panel and **urine dipstick**

    (3) Metabolic panel (e.g., calcium, thyroid function tests, cholesterol panel, fasting glucose)

  d. Electrocardiography. Evidence of a left atrial abnormality (LAA) or LVH signify cardiac damage, probably as a result of long-standing hypertension.

2. Additional studies may be indicated if secondary hypertension is suspected on the basis of the preliminary evaluation. Patients with a rapid deterioration of blood pressure control and those with very severe hypertension are also candidates for a work-up for secondary hypertension. (Table 23-2).

  a. Renal arterial disease

    (1) Angiotensin-converting enzyme (ACE) inhibitor challenge testing is usually the initial screening test of choice.

      (a) Test protocol. Patients should have normal sodium intake, no recent diuretic or ACE inhibitor intake, and no antihypertensive intake for 3 weeks prior (if possible). Isotropic renal blood flow and plasma renin activity (PRA) are tested before and 60 minutes after administration of captopril (25 mg orally) or enalapril (2.5 mg intravenously).

      (b) Test results. A positive test has an absolute increase in PRA of 10 ng/ml/hr or greater, a stimulated PRA of 12 ng/ml/hr or greater, a 150% or greater increase in PRA over the baseline, or a 20% or greater decrease in renal blood flow measured by isotopic renography.

    (2) Renal artery angiography is the invasive, gold-standard test for renal artery disease.

    (3) Other diagnostic tests for selected patients include renal vein renin levels, renal artery Doppler ultrasound, and magnetic resonance renal arteriography.

TABLE 23-2. Clinical Factors Associated with Diseases Causing Secondary Hypertension

Causative Diseases	Associated Clinical Factors
Renal arterial disease	Age of onset younger than 30 years or older than 50 years BP resistant to standard drug therapy Malignant hypertension Abdominal bruit, particularly if lateralized Renal dysfunction after administration of ACE inhibitors
Renal parenchymal disease	Elevated serum BUN and creatinine
Primary aldosteronism	Age of onset 30–50 years Symptoms of muscle weakness and paresthesia Unexplained hypokalemia (≤ 3.0 mEq/L) Hypernatremia (> 145 mEq/L)
Cushing's syndrome	Rapid weight gain Acne, hirsutism, moon facies, and purple striae Hyperglycemia Hypokalemia
Pheochromocytoma	Symptom triad: attacks of headaches, sweating, and palpitations BP resistant to standard drug therapy Pressor response to β blockers Family history of pheochromocytoma, medullary thyroid carcinoma, or hyperparathyroidism
Coarctation of the aorta	Symptoms of cold feet and leg claudication Arm BP $>$ leg BP Absent femoral artery pulses Systolic thrill in left posterior thorax Rib notching (i.e., increased collateral flow through intercostal arteries) and figure 3 sign (i.e., indentation of the aortic knob) on chest radiograph Bicuspid aortic valve as an associated congenital anomaly

ACE = angiotensin-converting enzyme; BP = blood pressure; BUN = blood urea nitrogen.

b. Renal parenchymal disease
   (1) Urinalysis
   (a) Red cell casts may be seen in patients with glomerulonephritis. White cell casts may occur in patients with pyelonephritis or interstitial nephritis. Fatty (lipid) casts may be present in patients with nephrotic syndrome.
   (b) Proteinuria may be seen in acute or chronic renal disease. If proteinuria is greater than 1+, then 24-hour urine protein levels should be measured to determine whether nephrotic syndrome is present.
   (2) Additional laboratory studies
   (a) Bacteriologic or serologic evidence of streptococcal infection indicates poststreptococcal glomerulonephritis.
   (b) Cytoplasmic antineutrophilic cytoplasmic antibody (C-ANCA) may indicate Wegener's granulomatosis, whereas perinuclear-ANCA (P-ANCA) may indicate polyarteritis nodosa.
   (c) Antinuclear antibodies (ANA) may indicate systemic lupus erythematosus (SLE).
   (d) Serum cryoglobulins indicate cryoglobulinemia that may be due to lymphoproliferative disorders (e.g., multiple myeloma), infections (e.g., hepatitis), or connective tissue diseases.
   (3) Renal ultrasound imaging. The kidneys are usually normal in patients with hypertension resulting from acute renal disease, whereas the kidneys are often small in patients with chronic renal disease.
   (4) Renal biopsy may be indicated to make a diagnosis.
c. Primary aldosteronism
   (1) Ratio of serum aldosterone to PRA is the first screening test and can help to distinguish essential hypertension from primary aldosteronism.
   (a) This ratio is usually greater than 400 in Conn's syndrome and bilateral adrenal hyperplasia.
   (b) This ratio is usually less than 200 in essential hypertension.
   (2) Aldosterone suppression test. A positive test shows that plasma aldosterone levels remain greater than 10 ng/dl (i.e., they "fail to suppress") after the intravenous administration of 2 L of normal saline over 4 hours.
   (3) Localization studies are important once primary aldosteronism is diagnosed. Abdominal computed tomography (CT) scans and adrenal vein aldosterone levels can help distinguish between adrenal adenoma

and bilateral adrenal hyperplasia as the cause of elevated aldosterone levels.

d. Cushing's syndrome

(1) Urinary free cortisol is the **initial screening test of choice.** A positive test showing more than 100 μg of cortisol in the 24-hour urine sample suggests Cushing's syndrome.

(2) Overnight dexamethasone suppression test. This inexpensive screening test is used if the urinary free cortisol test is abnormal. The test involves measuring a baseline plasma cortisol level in the morning, then administering 1 mg of dexamethasone orally at 11 PM, and repeating the cortisol measurement the following morning. In a positive test, the plasma cortisol is not suppressed below 5 μg/dl on the second morning.

(3) The high-dose dexamethasone suppression test can be used to confirm Cushing's syndrome when other tests are positive.

  (a) Test protocol. Measure the basal plasma cortisol and ACTH levels. Administer 0.5 mg of dexamethasone every 6 hours for 2 days followed by 2 mg every 6 hours for another 2 days. Measure urinary free cortisol and plasma cortisol on the second day after each dose level.

  (b) Test interpretation

   (i) Cushing's disease (ACTH-producing pituitary tumor leading to bilateral adrenal hyperplasia). Cortisol levels are suppressed to less than 50% of baseline levels by high-dose dexamethasone. ACTH levels are normal to elevated.

   (ii) Adrenal tumor. Cortisol levels are not suppressed, and ACTH levels are undetectable.

   (iii) Ectopic ACTH syndrome. Cortisol levels are not suppressed, and ACTH levels are elevated.

(4) CT or magnetic resonance imaging (MRI) scans of the adrenal glands can distinguish bilateral adrenal hyperplasia from adrenal adenomas.

e. Pheochromocytoma

(1) Urinary screening tests. Twenty-four-hour urine samples usually show elevated levels of **total catecholamines** (more than 150 μg/day), **vanillylmandelic acid** (more than 7 mg/day), and **metanephrine** (more than 1.3 mg/day) in cases of pheochromocytoma.

(2) Plasma catecholamine levels are increased in more than 90% of patients with pheochromocytoma.

      (3) Localization studies primarily include CT or MRI scans of the adrenal glands to identify the adrenal lesions.

    f. Coarctation of the aorta

      (1) Transthoracic echocardiography (TTE) is a useful initial screening test.

      (2) Aortography is the best test for confirming the diagnosis.

B. Treatment. Stable patients with stage 1–3 hypertension (see Table 23-1) are treated as outpatients with a combination of lifestyle modifications and pharmacologic agents (see Appendix B).

  1. Essential hypertension

    a. Lifestyle modifications may be initiated before drug therapy for patients with stage 1 hypertension. These modifications should be started concurrently with pharmacologic therapy for patients with more severe hypertension.

      (1) Lose weight if overweight.

      (2) Limit alcohol to 1 oz ethanol each day (e.g., 24 oz beer, 10 oz wine, or 2 oz 100-proof whiskey).

      (3) Increase aerobic physical activity.

      (4) Reduce dietary sodium to 2.5 g or less daily.

      (5) Maintain adequate dietary calcium, potassium, and **magnesium.**

      (6) Limit caffeine intake.

      (7) Stop smoking.

      (8) Reduce dietary fat and **cholesterol** for overall cardiac health.

    b. Pharmacologic therapy. Drug therapy is considered in patients with Stages 2–4 hypertension, those with hypertension refractory to lifestyle modifications, patients with coronary artery disease (CAD), and those with end-organ damage.

      (1) First-line agents have been proven to reduce mortality.

        (a) Diuretics [e.g., hydrochlorothiazide (25 mg daily)] are the least expensive agents and also provide synergistic antihypertensive effects when combined with other agents. Serum cholesterol and uric acid levels may increase.

        (b) β Blockers [e.g., metoprolol (25–50 mg twice daily), atenolol (25–50 mg daily)] are excellent antihypertensives and are particularly useful in patients who have previously had an MI.

      (2) Second-line agents can be considered if the patient has a contraindication to diuretic and β-blocker therapy or an associated condition (Table 23-3).

TABLE 23-3. Antihypertensive Agents That May be Considered for Common Associated Conditions

Associated Conditions	Recommended Agents	Contraindicated Agents
CAD	β Blockers, nitrates, amlodipine, diltiazem, or verapamil	Monotherapy with nifedipine or hydralazine
CHF (systolic)	ACE inhibitors or diuretics are first-line drugs; also newer calcium channel blockers (e.g., amlodipine, felodipine)	Nifedipine, diltiazem, and verapamil
Atrial fibrillation or flutter	β Blockers, diltiazem, or verapamil	Monotherapy with nifedipine or hydralazine
Diabetes mellitus	ACE inhibitors or ARBs	–
Benign prostatic hypertrophy	α-Adrenergic blockers (e.g., doxazosin, prazosin, terazosin)	–
Asthma	Calcium channel blockers or ACE inhibitors	β Blockers
Gout	–	Diuretics

ACE = angiotensin-converting enzyme; ARBs = angiotensin-receptor blockers; CAD = coronary artery disease; CHF = congestive heart failure; COPD = chronic obstructive pulmonary disease.

(a) **ACE inhibitors** are particularly useful for patients with left ventricular systolic dysfunction, prior MI, LVH, or diabetic nephropathy.

(b) **Calcium channel blockers** seem to be effective in patients with renal insufficiency. Nifedipine, diltiazem, and verapamil should generally be avoided in patients with left ventricular systolic dysfunction.

(c) **α-Adrenergic blockers** (e.g., doxazosin, prazosin, terazosin) can be considered in patients with benign prostatic hypertrophy.

(d) **Direct vasodilators** (e.g., hydralazine, minoxidil) can be helpful in patients with peripheral vascular disease.

HOT

KEY

> **Resistant hypertension** is diagnosed if the blood pressure remains greater than 140/90 mm Hg despite adequate compliance with lifestyle modifications and drug therapy with three agents at near-maximal doses. In this situation, consider non-adherence to drug therapy, secondary causes of hypertension, associated conditions (e.g., chronic pain, renal insufficiency), volume overload owing to CHF or renal dysfunction, or "white-coat" hypertension (i.e., hypertension that is only present during periods of anxiety).

2. **Secondary hypertension.** Treatment usually requires appropriate subspecialty consultation.
   a. **Renal arterial disease**
      (1) **Surgical revascularization** is the most reliable therapy for atherosclerotic disease. Balloon angioplasty may be indicated for unilateral short diseased segments, but restenosis rates are higher than with surgical correction.
      (2) **Renal artery balloon angioplasty** is the preferred treatment for fibromuscular dysplasia.
      (3) **Medical therapy** is reserved for those patients who are poor candidates for revascularization. Antihypertensive therapy includes calcium channel blockers, β blockers, and diuretics; ACE inhibitors should be avoided.
   b. **Renal parenchymal disease**
      (1) **Acute renal disease.** Therapy is aimed at correcting the primary disorder and providing supportive care.
      (2) **Chronic renal disease**
         (a) **Loop diuretics** (e.g., furosemide 20–80 mg orally one to four times daily) may be used to maintain normal volume status.
         (b) **Calcium channel blockers, labetalol,** and **minoxidil** may be useful antihypertensive agents.
         (c) **Hemodialysis** or **renal transplantation** may help control blood pressure in patients with end-stage renal disease.
   c. **Primary aldosteronism**
      (1) **Adrenal tumors** are treated with surgical excision. Seventy-five percent of patients are cured; twenty-five percent remain hypertensive and require drug therapy.
      (2) **Adrenal hyperplasia** may be treated medically with **spironolactone** (25–100 mg orally every 8 hours). Surgery is indicated for patients with a condition that is refractory to medical therapy.

d. Cushing's syndrome
  (1) Adrenal tumors are treated with adrenalectomy.
  (2) Adrenal hyperplasia can be treated with total adrenalectomy. Alternatively, a "medical adrenalectomy" may be accomplished by administering medications that inhibit steroid synthesis, such as ketoconazole (600–1200 mg daily), mitotane (2–3 g daily), or metyrapone (2–3 g daily).
  (3) Pituitary adenomas are treated with transphenoidal microsurgical tumor removal. If the patient remains symptomatic, then bilateral adrenalectomy or "medical adrenalectomy" can be considered.

e. Pheochromocytoma
  (1) Medical therapy involves primarily α-adrenergic blockade with phenoxybenzamine (usually 10–50 mg orally twice daily). β Blockers can be added after α blockade has been established.
  (2) Surgical therapy, the definitive treatment, involves removal of the tumor with careful perioperative hemodynamic monitoring.

f. Coarctation of the aorta
  (1) Medical therapy may include β blockers, ACE inhibitors, or calcium channel blockers.
  (2) Surgical therapy with resection of the narrow aortic segment followed by end-to-end anastomosis is the treatment of choice.

References

Gifford RW: Treatment of patients with systemic arterial hypertension. In *Hurst's the Heart,* 9th ed. Edited by Alexander RW, Schlant RC, Fuster V. New York, McGraw-Hill, 1998, pp 1673–1695.

Hall WD: Diagnostic evaluation of the patient with systemic arterial hypertension. In *Hurst's the Heart,* 9th ed. Edited by Alexander RW, Schlant RC, Fuster V. New York, McGraw-Hill, 1998, pp 1651–1672.

Schwartz GL, Sheps SG: A review of the sixth report of the Joint National Committee on prevention, detection, evaluation, and treatment of high blood pressure. *Curr Opin Cardiol* 14(2):161–168, 1999.

The sixth report of the Joint National Committee on prevention, detection, evaluation, and treatment of high blood pressure. *Arch Intern Med* 157:2413–2446, 1997.

24. Pulmonary Hypertension

▮ I ▮ INTRODUCTION

A. **Pulmonary hypertension** is diagnosed when pulmonary artery pressures exceed 30/15 mm Hg and there is clinical, radiographic, electrocardiographic, or echocardiographic evidence of increased pulmonary pressures.

B. **Untreated severe pulmonary hypertension** carries a high mortality rate, but identification and treatment of reversible causes may improve the survival rate for some patients.

▮ II ▮ CAUSES OF PULMONARY HYPERTENSION

A. **Primary causes.** Primary pulmonary hypertension (i.e., plexogenic pulmonary arteriopathy) is a disorder of the pulmonary arteries themselves. This type of pulmonary hypertension is most common in young women who present with right-sided heart failure. Most patients have a rapidly downhill course, with an average survival of less than 3 years. Primary pulmonary hypertension can be diagnosed only after secondary causes have been excluded. Primary pulmonary hypertension is less common and more difficult to treat than secondary pulmonary hypertension.

B. **Secondary causes.** When increased pulmonary artery pressures are caused by increased pressure "downstream" (or beyond the pulmonary capillaries), the hypertension is called **postcapillary pulmonary hypertension.** When the increased pulmonary pressures result from abnormalities "upstream" or within the pulmonary capillaries, the hypertension is called **precapillary/capillary pulmonary hypertension.**

  1. **Postcapillary causes**

    a. **Increased left ventricular pressure.** Disorders include:

      (1) Systolic or diastolic left ventricular dysfunction (most common)

      (2) Aortic stenosis

      (3) Constrictive pericarditis

    b. **Increased left atrial pressure with normal left ventricular pressure.** Disorders include:

      (1) Mitral stenosis

      (2) Left atrial myxoma

      (3) Cor triatriatum

    c. Pulmonary veno-occlusive disease. Fibrotic changes in the veins or venules are of unclear etiology but may be associated with:

      (1) Malignancy

      (2) Chemotherapy

      (3) Bone marrow transplantation

2. Precapillary/capillary causes

    a. Chronic obstructive pulmonary disease (COPD)

    b. Restrictive lung disease

    c. Vascular disease (i.e., small vessel occlusion)

      (1) Vasculitis

      (2) Pulmonary emboli

      (3) Schistosomiasis

    d. Miscellaneous causes

      (1) Hypoxia

      (2) Acidosis

      (3) Polycythemia

      (4) Hepatic cirrhosis

      (5) Intracardiac left-to-right shunt [via atrial septal defect (ASD) or ventricular septal defect (VSD)]

      (6) Sleep apnea

HOT
▶
KEY

Sleep apnea is increasingly being recognized as a cause of hypoxia leading to secondary pulmonary hypertension.

III CLINICAL MANIFESTATIONS OF PULMONARY HYPERTENSION

A. Symptoms may include:

1. Dyspnea
2. Chest pain (partially as a result of right ventricular ischemia)
3. Fatigue
4. Syncope or near syncope
5. Peripheral edema (from right ventricular failure)

B. Signs. Patients with pulmonary hypertension often present with physical examination findings that reflect **right ventricular failure.** The following findings are typical:

1. Increased jugular venous pressure
2. A right ventricular lift
3. A right-sided third heart sound (S_3) or fourth heart sound (S_4)
4. Accentuated pulmonary component of the second heart sound (P_2) that is louder than the aortic component of the second heart sound (A_2)

5. Murmurs of tricuspid and pulmonic valve regurgitation

6. Hepatomegaly and ascites

7. Peripheral cyanosis and edema

HOT KEY

Evidence of right ventricular failure almost always indicates pulmonary hypertension.

IV Approach to the Patient

A. Preliminary evaluation

1. Physical examination

a. Carefully compare the second heart sound intensity in the left second interspace (P_2) to that in the right second interspace (A_2). A P_2 that is louder than the A_2 suggests increased pulmonary pressures.

b. Assess for a left-sided S_3 or S_4 gallop, which may indicate left ventricular dysfunction (i.e., a postcapillary etiology). Also, listen for murmurs and extra heart sounds that may indicate valvular stenosis (i.e., mitral or aortic) or a left atrial myxoma, respectively.

2. Laboratory studies

a. Polycythemia is often present with chronic hypoxia.

b. Arterial blood gas sampling is indicated.

3. Electrocardiography. The electrocardiogram (ECG) usually shows right axis deviation (RAD). Right atrial enlargement, right ventricular hypertrophy (RVH), and right bundle branch block (RBBB) are also common findings.

4. Chest radiography

a. Pulmonary hypertension from all etiologies will usually result in enlarged central pulmonary arteries visible on the chest radiograph. Right atrial and ventricular enlargement may also be seen in severe cases.

b. Evidence of the underlying cause may be evident radiographically. For example:

(1) In emphysema, there may be "pruning" of the distal vessels, hyperinflation, or flat diaphragms.

(2) In left ventricular dysfunction, there may be left atrial enlargement, ventricular enlargement, or both, or evidence of pulmonary edema.

(3) In mitral or aortic stenosis, valvular calcification may be noted.

B. Confirmatory testing. Many noninvasive and invasive diagnostic tests may be used to further define the cause and severity of the patient's pulmonary hypertension. Testing to exclude cardiac causes of postcapillary pulmonary hypertension is indicated. Obtaining tests in the following order is a reasonable approach in the work-up of pulmonary hypertension in a stable patient.

1. **Echocardiography**
   a. **Two-dimensional and Doppler echocardiography**
      (1) The pulmonary artery pressure can be estimated.
      (2) RVH, right ventricular enlargement, paradoxical motion of the interventricular septum (suggesting increased right ventricular pressure or volume), and right atrial enlargement may accompany pulmonary hypertension.
      (3) Left ventricular dysfunction, mitral stenosis, aortic stenosis, or left atrial myxoma suggests a diagnosis of postcapillary pulmonary hypertension.
   b. **Bubble study.** A bubble study allows detection of an intracardiac shunt.
2. **Pulmonary function testing**
   a. A decreased diffusing capacity of the lungs for carbon monoxide (DLCO) and a mild restrictive defect are common findings regardless of the cause of pulmonary hypertension.
   b. Severe obstructive disease in a smoker is the most helpful finding because it usually establishes COPD as the diagnosis.
3. **Ventilation-perfusion (V/Q) lung scanning.** If no cause of postcapillary hypertension or COPD has been found, evaluation for chronic thromboembolism is usually necessary.
4. **Sleep studies** are usually indicated in patients with risk factors for sleep apnea (i.e., male sex, obesity, and a history of snoring). Sleep studies, however, do not correlate well with the degree of pulmonary hypertension and may lead to false-positive results.
5. **Right heart catheterization.** If the diagnosis is still elusive, invasive testing with right heart catheterization using a Swan-Ganz catheter may be indicated to measure right heart pressures and determine cardiac output (CO).
   a. Right heart catheterization can distinguish accurately between precapillary/capillary pulmonary hypertension [which has a normal pulmonary capillary wedge pressure (PCWP)] and postcapillary pulmonary hypertension (which has an increased PCWP).
   b. A **pulmonary angiogram** can also be performed to evaluate possible pulmonary embolic disease.
   c. Leaving the Swan-Ganz catheter in the pulmonary artery may guide vasodilator therapy in the coronary care unit (CCU).

V TREATMENT

A. Primary pulmonary hypertension

1. **Oxygen therapy** decreases pulmonary vasoconstriction in hypoxic patients (oxygen saturation < 90%), slowing the progression of pulmonary hypertension.

2. **Pharmacologic therapy** of right-sided heart failure is guided by the patient's symptoms.

   a. **Salt restriction and diuretics** reduce peripheral edema and hepatic congestion.

   b. **Digoxin therapy** is controversial because it may increase pulmonary vascular resistance. Some authorities recommend its use to improve right ventricular function.

   c. **Vasodilator therapy** is useful to reduce pulmonary vascular resistance. Therapy should be instituted in a CCU with a Swan-Ganz catheter in place to document the response of pulmonary artery pressures and the CO.

      (1) **Prostacyclin** and **adenosine** are most commonly used as screening agents to identify patients likely to respond to chronic vasodilator therapy.

      (2) **Oral systemic vasodilators** (e.g., calcium channel blockers, α-adrenergic blockers, hydralazine, and nitrates) can be tried during a "vasodilator trial" with a pulmonary artery catheter in place.

      (3) **Chronic intravenous prostacyclin** (e.g., epoprostenol 2–16 ng/kg/min) has been shown to improve mortality and morbidity in patients with severe primary pulmonary hypertension and is usually instituted while they are awaiting transplantation.

   d. **Anticoagulation therapy**

      (1) Treatment with warfarin or antiplatelet agents is generally recommended because of the high incidence of in situ thrombosis in the pulmonary vasculature due to endothelial injury. Caution is indicated in patients with syncope.

      (2) Routine prophylaxis with subcutaneous heparin is advisable during hospitalization or prolonged periods of immobility.

3. **Heart-lung and lung transplantation** can be considered in suitable candidates with end-stage disease.

B. Secondary pulmonary hypertension

1. **General measures**

   a. **Oxygen therapy** should be instituted to treat hypoxia. More than 15 hours of nasal canula oxygen per day has a long-term mortality benefit in hypoxic patients with COPD.

   b. **Phlebotomy.** Patients showing polycythemia with a

hematocrit that exceeds 60% may benefit from phlebotomy to reduce blood viscosity.

   c. Salt restriction, diuretics, and sometimes **digoxin** are used to treat cor pulmonale.

2. Specific measures. Treatment is aimed at the underlying disease.

   a. Congestive heart failure (CHF) management is discussed in Chapter 16 IV.

   b. COPD can be treated with smoking cessation, bronchodilators, inhaled and systemic steroids, theophylline, and oxygen therapy when appropriate.

   c. Thromboembolic disease is treated with chronic anticoagulation therapy. Thromboembolectomy is often considered for patients who develop pulmonary hypertension as a result of major pulmonary artery occlusion.

   d. Sleep apnea can be improved by weight reduction, avoidance of alcohol and sedatives, and nighttime oxygen with or without continuous positive airway pressure.

References

Gaine SP, Rubin LJ: Primary pulmonary hypertension. *Lancet* 352:719–725, 1998.

Herner SJ, Mauro LS: Epoprostenol in primary pulmonary hypertension. *Ann Pharmacother* 33(3):340–347, 1999.

McLaughlin VV, Rich S: Pulmonary hypertension: Advances in medical and surgical interventions. *J Heart Lung Transplant* 17:739–743, 1998.

Moraes D, Loscalzo J: Pulmonary hypertension: Newer concepts in diagnosis and management. *Clin Cardiol* 20:676–682, 1997.

Ricciardi MJ, Rubenfire M: How to manage secondary pulmonary hypertension. *Postgrad Med* 105(2):183–190, 1999.

PART VIII

OTHER CAUSES
OF HEART DISEASE

25. Congenital Heart Disease in Adults

INTRODUCTION

A. Incidence. Congenital heart disease occurs in roughly 8 of 1000 live births in the United States. Almost one-third of these patients are severely affected and subsequently need surgical correction.

B. Definitions. The most common congenital heart disorders are described:

    1. A **ventricular septal defect (VSD)** is an opening in the ventricular septum between the left and right ventricles.

    2. An **atrial septal defect (ASD)** is an opening in the atrial septum between the left and right atria.

> **HOT KEY**
>
> An ASD should be distinguished from a patent foramen ovale (PFO). A PFO may persist into adulthood in as many as 15% of patients.

    3. Patent ductus arteriosus (PDA) is the persistent patency of the vessel that connects the pulmonary artery to the aorta in the fetus.

    4. Coarctation of the aorta is a discrete narrowing of the aortic arch, typically just distal to the takeoff of the left subclavian artery.

    5. Pulmonic stenosis is narrowing of the pulmonic valve. This disorder is discussed in Chapter 19.

C. Epidemiology

    1. Nearly one-third of patients with congenital heart disease have a VSD. An ASD, PDA, coarctation of the aorta, and pulmonic stenosis account for most other cases.

    2. Among patients with congenital heart disease who survive into adulthood, almost one-third have an ASD.

3. Congenital heart disease accounts for about 2% of cases of heart disease in adults.

D. Prognosis. With improved detection and treatment, many infants with congenital heart disease survive into adulthood. An understanding of the complications associated with uncorrected congenital heart disease, as well as surveillance care for patients who have undergone surgical therapy is essential.

II VENTRICULAR SEPTAL DEFECT (VSD)

A. Anatomic types
  1. **Paramembranous VSDs** are the most common type of VSD and involve the membranous portion of the ventricular septum.
  2. Less common types include:
     a. **Apical muscular defects** (involving the muscular septum at the ventricular apex)
     b. **Inlet defects** (occurring beneath the septal leaflet of the tricuspid valve)
     c. **Outlet defects** (involving the left ventricular outflow tract)
B. Natural history
  1. Most VSDs are small and, therefore, do not cause significant medical problems. In fact, 50% of small VSDs close spontaneously by 1 year of age, and 90% close by 8 years of age.
  2. Moderate-sized VSDs are usually diagnosed early in infancy. Many patients will develop congestive heart failure (CHF), which resolves after spontaneous or surgical closure of the VSD.
  3. Large VSDs usually cause CHF, requiring 80% of affected infants to be hospitalized by 4 months of age. Without surgical correction, most of these patients will die in early childhood.
C. Abnormal physiology
  1. The larger the VSD, the greater is the flow of blood from the left ventricle to the right ventricle.
  2. In large VSDs, both pulmonary blood flow and pulmonary vascular resistance increase. If pulmonary vascular resistance continues to increase, the left-to-right shunt may reverse direction. The ensuing right-to-left shunt may cause cyanosis and clubbing accompanied by biventricular failure (i.e., **Eisenmenger's syndrome).**
D. Approach to the patient
  1. **History.** The severity of the patient's symptoms depends on the size of the VSD and the degree of pulmonary hypertension.
     a. **Infants** may present with difficulty breathing, grunting respirations, and fatigue, particularly during feedings. These infants are usually underweight.

      b. Young adults may complain of dyspnea on exertion and orthopnea.

  2. Cardiac examination

      a. Palpation

         (1) A systolic thrill at the left lower sternal border is common.

         (2) A right ventricular lift may signify right ventricular dysfunction and pulmonary hypertension.

      b. Heart sounds

         (1) As the pulmonary artery pressures increase, the intensity of the pulmonary component of the second heart sound (P_2) increases and the second heart sound (S_2) progressively becomes more narrowly split.

         (2) A third heart sound (S_3) may signify right or left ventricular systolic dysfunction or both.

      c. Murmurs

         (1) Large shunts generate a loud, harsh holosystolic murmur that is best heard at the left sternal border in the third and fourth interspaces.

         (2) Pulmonary hypertension may be accompanied by the murmurs of pulmonic or tricuspid regurgitation.

  3. Electrocardiogram (ECG)

      a. The ECG may appear normal in patients with a small VSD.

      b. With larger shunts and the development of pulmonary hypertension, the ECG may show right, left, or biventricular hypertrophy.

  4. Chest radiograph

      a. The chest radiograph may show evidence of right or left ventricular hypertrophy (LVH) and left atrial enlargement.

      b. If pulmonary vascular disease develops, the pulmonary artery may be dilated with diminished distal vascularity.

  5. Echocardiogram

      a. Echocardiography can be used to evaluate right and left ventricular size and function.

      b. Doppler ultrasound imaging can also be used to estimate the size of the shunt and the pulmonary artery pressure.

  6. Cardiac catheterization can definitively diagnose a VSD by detecting an increase (or "step-up") in the oxygen saturation from the right atrium to the right ventricle. Oxygen saturation measurements can be used to calculate the ratio of pulmonary-to-systemic blood flow (Qp/Qs). Left ventriculography can be used to show the interventricular shunt.

E. Treatment

  1. Medical therapy is recommended for patients with a small shunt (i.e., a Qp/Qs < 1.5).

      a. Diuretics and **vasodilator agents** [e.g., angiotensin-converting enzyme (ACE) inhibitors, hydralazine] can improve the signs and symptoms of CHF by reducing the magnitude of the left-to-right shunt.

b. Antibiotic prophylaxis is recommended for all patients with an uncorrected VSD to prevent bacterial endocarditis (see Chapter 22).

2. Surgical therapy is recommended for asymptomatic infants without spontaneous closure by 3–5 years of age and also for adults with a significant left-to-right shunt (i.e., a Qp/Qs ≥ 1.5).

HOT KEY

Surgery is contraindicated in patients with severe pulmonary artery hypertension or Eisenmenger's syndrome because it may exacerbate right ventricular failure.

---

a. Surgery has an operative mortality rate of less than 3%. Complete heart block occurs in less than 2% of cases.

b. Antibiotic prophylaxis is recommended for 6 months following the surgical closure of a VSD (see Chapter 22).

III ATRIAL SEPTAL DEFECT (ASD)

A. Anatomic types

1. Ostium secundum ASDs are the most common type, accounting for more than two-thirds of all ASDs. The defect at the **fossa ovalis** affects the middle portion of the atrial septum.

2. Ostium primum ASDs are less common, affecting the lower portion of the atrial septum.

3. Sinus venosus ASDs are least common, affecting the upper portion of the atrial septum. An associated condition may be anomalous pulmonary veins, which empty into the right atrium or superior vena cava.

B. Natural history

1. In patients with a mild ASD, the degree of left-to-right shunting is small, and the mild increase in pulmonary blood flow is well tolerated. It is rare for a secundum ASD to spontaneously close after 2 years of age.

2. In patients with a large shunt, pulmonary hypertension is usually mild. Symptoms usually begin when patients are in their late teens or twenties.

3. Severe pulmonary hypertension, complicated by right-sided heart failure and right-to-left shunting, occurs in less than 15% of young adults.

4. Patients with large uncorrected ASDs frequently die in their forties or fifties. Some patients, however, may survive to old age if pulmonary hypertension does not occur.

      a. CHF is the most common cause of death in patients with uncorrected ASDs who are older than 40 years.

      b. Other causes of morbidity and mortality include pulmonary embolism, infection, and complications of atrial flutter or fibrillation.

   5. Infective endocarditis is very rare in patients with secundum ASDs.

C. Abnormal physiology

   1. The larger the ASD, the greater is the flow of blood from the left atrium to the right atrium.

   2. In large ASDs, the pulmonary blood flow increases while the pulmonary vascular resistance remains approximately the same. Eisenmenger's syndrome rarely develops.

D. Approach to the patient

   1. History

      a. Whereas most patients with small or moderate shunts remain asymptomatic, young adults with large left-to-right shunts may report dyspnea on exertion and fatigue.

      b. Palpitations may indicate supraventricular or ventricular arrhythmias.

   2. Cardiac examination

      a. Palpation may demonstrate a right ventricular lift.

      b. Heart sounds

         (1) The S_2 is widely split and does not vary with respiration (i.e., a fixed split S_2).

         (2) The intensity of the P_2 may be accentuated, even in the absence of pulmonary hypertension.

      c. Murmurs. The increased right ventricular stroke volume results in a systolic ejection murmur in the second interspace at the left sternal border.

   3. ECG. The ECG commonly shows evidence of right atrial enlargement, right ventricular hypertrophy (RVH), or incomplete or complete right bundle branch block (RBBB).

   4. Chest radiograph. The chest radiograph characteristically shows mild-to-moderate enlargement of the cardiac silhouette and the branch pulmonary arteries.

   5. Echocardiogram

      a. Two-dimensional echocardiography (2DE) can show evidence of right ventricular volume overload.

      b. Doppler ultrasound imaging can allow visualization of the shunt and estimation of the pulmonary artery pressure.

      c. A **bubble study,** which is the injection of an agitated saline into a peripheral vein during echocardiographic imaging, can usually detect an ASD.

   6. Cardiac catheterization can definitively diagnose an ASD by detecting a "step-up" in the oxygen saturation from the superior and inferior vena cavae to the right atrium. Oxygen saturation measurements can be used to calculate the ratio of pulmonary to systemic blood flow. Right atrial angiography can be used to show the interatrial shunt.

E. Treatment

    1. Observation is appropriate for asymptomatic patients with a small shunt (i.e, a Qp/Qs < 1.5).

    2. Antibiotic prophylaxis is used to prevent bacterial endocarditis in patients with ostium primum and sinus venosus ASDs. It is not necessary, however, for patients with an isolated secundum ASD (see Chapter 22).

    3. Surgical therapy

        a. Surgical closure (e.g., direct suture or patch) is recommended for symptomatic patients as well as asymptomatic patients with a Qp/Qs of 1.5 or greater.

        b. Transcatheter closure (e.g., double-umbrella clamshell or buttoned device) is currently under investigation as a promising nonsurgical procedure for ASD closure.

HOT

KEY

Closure of an ASD is contraindicated in patients with severe pulmonary artery hypertension with a reversed (right-to-left) shunt because of the risk of acute right-sided heart failure.

IV PATENT DUCTUS ARTERIOSUS (PDA)

A. Natural history

    1. A small shunt through a PDA does not usually reduce life expectancy, although the risk of endocarditis is increased.

    2. In patients with a moderate or large PDA, CHF, pulmonary hypertension, and endocarditis may occur. Premature death can be expected in the patient's late teens or early adulthood if the PDA is not surgically corrected.

B. Abnormal physiology

    1. The left-to-right shunt from the aorta to the pulmonary artery leads to an increase in both pulmonary and left ventricular blood flow and pulmonary vascular resistance.

        a. Left ventricular dilatation and failure may develop as a result of increased left ventricular flow.

        b. Obliterative changes in the pulmonary vasculature may lead to pulmonary hypertension.

    2. The left-to-right shunt into the pulmonary artery may also serve as a nidus for infection, predisposing the patient to both a mycotic aneurysm and multiple pulmonary emboli.

C. Approach to the patient
1. History
    a. Many patients with a PDA were born prematurely. Exposure to rubella in the first trimester also places the fetus at an increased risk for developing a PDA.

    b. Patients typically remain asymptomatic until left ventricular dysfunction or pulmonary hypertension develops. Dyspnea and fatigue in an infant or child may signify these complications.

2. Cardiac examination
    a. Peripheral pulses are usually bounding, reflecting the low diastolic blood pressure and wide pulse pressure, which result from the diastolic runoff from the aorta to the pulmonary artery.

    b. Palpation of the precordium may demonstrate a hyperdynamic impulse, which is displaced in patients with large shunts. A continuous thrill is occasionally present.

    c. Murmurs. Classically, a PDA generates a **continuous, rough "machinery" murmur** that is best heard at the left upper sternal border. This murmur may peak near the S_2.

3. ECG
    a. Left atrial abnormality (LAA) and LVH are common findings.

    b. RVH may signify the presence of pulmonary hypertension.

4. Chest radiograph
    a. In patients with large shunts, the left atrium and ventricle may be enlarged.

    b. In older patients with Eisenmenger's syndrome, the central pulmonary arteries may be enlarged with tapering of the vasculature in the lung periphery.

5. Echocardiogram
    a. 2DE can show left atrial and ventricular enlargement.

    b. Doppler ultrasound imaging can be used to estimate the size of the shunt from the aorta to the pulmonary artery, as well as to measure the pulmonary artery pressure.

6. Cardiac catheterization
is important in confirming the diagnosis. A "step-up" in oxygen saturation from the right ventricle to the pulmonary artery supports the diagnosis. Aortography can be used to demonstrate the magnitude of the shunt by opacifying the ductus and pulmonary arteries.

D. Treatment
1. Medical therapy
    a. Indomethacin is often used in infants to close the PDA, which is believed to be kept open by prostaglandins. Some cases, however, are resistant to this treatment.

    b. Diuretics, digoxin, and **ACE inhibitors** may be considered for patients with CHF.

    c. Antibiotic prophylaxis is recommended for patients before, and for 6 months following, surgical correction (see Chapter 22).

  2. Surgical correction is recommended for infants with a PDA that is resistant to indomethacin treatment and for those who are older than 1 year.

    a. Surgical closure of the PDA is safe (mortality rate $< 0.5\%$) and may involve suture ligation or patch closure.

    b. Transcatheter closure using either a double-umbrella clamshell or coil closure has shown promise but is still experimental.

V COARCTATION OF THE AORTA

A. Natural history

  1. Most patients with coarctation of the aorta present with CHF early in infancy.

  2. Without corrective surgery, many patients will develop severe hypertension, aortic rupture, or intracranial hemorrhage in their twenties or thirties. CHF may also develop because of hypertensive heart disease. The average age of death for patients surviving childhood without surgical correction is roughly 35 years.

B. Abnormal physiology

  1. LVH develops from increased resistance due to the coarctation. Left ventricular dilatation and failure may result eventually.

  2. Collateral vessels develop through the intercostal arteries to supply blood to the lower extremities.

C. Approach to the patient

  1. History

    a. Infants may have difficulty breathing and poor weight gain.

    b. Children and young adults may report dyspnea, fatigue, or symptoms of leg claudication when running.

  2. Cardiac examination

    a. Vital signs. Hypertension is present in the upper extremities, but the blood pressure is low or normal in the lower extremities. A difference of more than 15 mm Hg in the systolic blood pressure between the upper and lower extremities should raise the suspicion of aortic coarctation.

    b. Peripheral pulses

      (1) Strong pulsations are present in the carotid arteries.

      (2) The femoral pulses are weak and delayed compared with the brachial or radial pulses. The patient's feet are often cold.

    c. Heart sounds. A fourth heart sound (S_4) is frequently present owing to diastolic dysfunction associated with severe hypertension.

  d. Murmurs

    (1) A late systolic ejection blowing murmur from the coarct is typically heard posteriorly between the scapulae. A continuous, low-pitched murmur over the chest wall may occur because of the collateral circulation.

    (2) Because one-third of patients with aortic coarctation have an associated bicuspid aortic valve, the murmur of aortic stenosis, regurgitation, or both may be present.

3. ECG. LAA and LVH may be present.

4. Chest radiograph (Figure 25-1)

  a. The heart size is usually at the upper limits of normal.

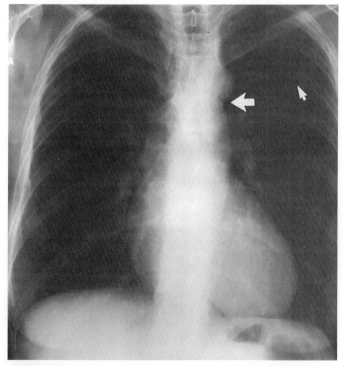

FIGURE 25-1. Posteroanterior chest radiograph of a patient with coarctation of the aorta showing the figure 3 sign (*large arrow*) of the deformed descending aorta. Areas of rib notching can be appreciated (*small arrow*). (Courtesy of C. Colangelo, M.D., San Francisco, CA)

    b. Rib notching may be observed because of increased collateral flow through intercostal arteries. This is usually not seen in patients younger than 7 years.

    c. The **figure 3 sign** represents the dilated aorta above the coarctation, the central indentation from the coarct itself, and the poststenotic dilatation just below the coarct.

  5. Echocardiogram

    a. 2DE is useful in assessing left ventricular size and function.

    b. Imaging of the aorta may allow visualization of the aortic coarctation.

  6. Cardiac catheterization can demonstrate left ventricular hypertension and a drop in pressure in the descending aorta. Aortography can demonstrate the exact location and extent of the aortic coarctation.

D. Treatment

  1. Medical therapy consists mainly of antihypertensive agents, including β blockers, ACE inhibitors, and calcium channel blockers.

  2. Surgical therapy

    a. Surgical resection of the coarctation is recommended for patients younger than 20 years.

    b. For patients between 20 and 40 years, surgery should be considered for those with severe hypertension. Unfortunately, roughly 25% of patients who undergo surgical correction will continue to have hypertension.

    c. Because the surgical risk increases significantly with age, surgical correction is controversial in patients older than 50 years.

References

Brickner ME, Hillis LD, Lange RA: Congenital heart disease in adults. *N Engl J Med* 342:256–263, 334–342, 2000.

Connelly MS, Webb GD, Somerville J, et al: Canadian Consensus Conference on Adult Congenital Heart Disease. *Can J Cardiol* 14:395–452, 1998.

Deanfield JE, Gersh BJ, Warnes CA, et al: Congenital heart disease in adults. In *Hurst's the Heart,* 9th ed. Edited by Alexander RW, Schlant RC, Fuster V. New York, McGraw-Hill, 1998, pp 1995–2027.

Foster E: Congenital heart disease in adults. *Western J Med* 163:492–498, 1995.

Somerville J: Management of adults with congenital heart disease: an increasing problem. *Ann Rev Med* 48:283–293, 1997.

26. Systemic Diseases

I **INTRODUCTION.** Systemic diseases [e.g., alcohol abuse, diabetes mellitus, acquired immune deficiency syndrome (AIDS), rheumatologic and connective tissue diseases, renal diseases, thyroid diseases, and neoplastic diseases] may be associated with a wide spectrum of cardiovascular disorders (e.g., cardiomyopathy, pericarditis).

II **ALCOHOL ABUSE.** Chronic alcohol abuse is associated with several life-threatening cardiovascular disorders.

A. Cardiomyopathy refers to ventricular dysfunction that results from a variety of disorders [e.g., congestive heart failure (CHF)].
  1. Alcohol abuse is responsible for almost one-third of the cases of cardiomyopathy that are referred to heart failure centers. Patients typically have dilated cardiomyopathy with four-chamber enlargement.
  2. CHF most commonly occurs in middle-aged men who have abused alcohol for at least 10 years, although women may also be affected.
  3. Abstinence may improve ventricular function in some patients. Survival rates are roughly 80% higher among those patients with CHF who abstain from alcohol compared with those who continue drinking.
B. Arrhythmias. Alcoholic binges increase levels of plasma catecholamines tenfold, which may precipitate arrhythmias.
  1. **Atrial arrhythmias.** Patients who have recently consumed large amounts of alcohol may develop **holiday heart syndrome** (i.e, a sudden onset of atrial fibrillation, atrial flutter, or other supraventricular tachycardia). This syndrome most commonly occurs during a hospital admission for alcohol withdrawal.
  2. **Ventricular arrhythmias** (e.g., ventricular tachycardia and fibrillation) commonly occur in patients with alcoholic cardiomyopathy, contributing to an increase in sudden death.
C. Hypertension. Both social drinking and heavy drinking are associated with an increase in blood pressure, which is largely attributable to an increase in peripheral vascular resistance. Hypertension in actively drinking patients is less responsive to antihypertensive medication.
D. Coronary artery disease (CAD). The quantity of alcohol inges-

tion, rather than alcohol type (e.g., beer, wine, whiskey), is the more important predictor of cardiovascular risk.

1. **Mild alcohol use** may be associated with elevated levels of high-density lipoproteins (HDLs) and, subsequently, a decreased risk for CAD.
2. **Heavy alcohol use** is consistently associated with high mortality rates from cardiovascular disease and cancer.

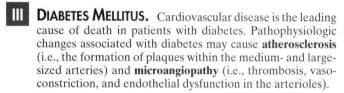 **DIABETES MELLITUS.** Cardiovascular disease is the leading cause of death in patients with diabetes. Pathophysiologic changes associated with diabetes may cause **atherosclerosis** (i.e., the formation of plaques within the medium- and large-sized arteries) and **microangiopathy** (i.e., thrombosis, vasoconstriction, and endothelial dysfunction in the arterioles).

A. **CAD**
1. Coronary atherosclerosis tends to be more severe in patients with diabetes compared with those who do not have diabetes.
2. The risk of myocardial infarction (MI) is three times higher in patients with diabetes compared with those who do not have diabetes.
3. Because the small distal branches of the coronary circulation are often diffusely diseased, revascularization options may be limited.

HOT
KEY

In some patients with diabetes, an autonomic neuropathy may result in cardiac denervation. These patients should be carefully monitored for silent ischemia, which is the onset of myocardial ischemia or infarction without the typical symptom of chest pain.

B. **CHF** is common in patients with diabetes. CHF may occur as a result of myocardia ischemia or infarction from coronary atherosclerosis, hypertension, or microangiopathy.
C. **Cerebral and peripheral vascular disease** commonly occur in patients with diabetes and primarily affect the smaller arteries.
D. **Hypertension** is more common in patients with diabetes compared with the general population. Causes include impaired compliance of large arteries, atherosclerosis of the renal arteries, endothelial proliferation of the renal arterioles, and abnormalities of the renin-angiotensin system.
E. **Arrhythmias.** Diabetic neuropathy may affect the sympathetic and parasympathetic nervous systems, resulting in a variety of atrial or ventricular tachyarrhythmias.

IV ACQUIRED IMMUNE DEFICIENCY SYNDROME (AIDS)

is caused by the human immunodeficiency virus type-1 (HIV-1). While pulmonary, gastrointestinal, and neurologic complications from AIDS are more common, cardiac involvement also occurs. Cardiac disorders may result from HIV-1 itself, opportunistic infections, or malignancy.

A. Pericardial disease (e.g., pericardial effusion and pericarditis) is common in patients with AIDS.

  1. Incidence. Pericardial effusion occurs in roughly 20% of patients with AIDS. While most cases are asymptomatic, roughly 10% of those with effusion may develop tamponade each year.

  2. Causes. The causes of AIDS-related pericardial effusion and pericarditis are broad and include malignancy (e.g., Kaposi's sarcoma, non-Hodgkin's lymphoma) and infection (bacterial, viral, fungal, and protozoal).

B. Myocardial disease commonly leads to death in patients with AIDS.

  1. Myocarditis refers to myocardial inflammation that may lead to myocardial scarring and systolic dysfunction. Patients usually present with chest pain, elevated cardiac serum enzyme levels, and ventricular dysfunction.

    a. Incidence. As many as 50% of all patients with AIDS have some degree of myocarditis during the course of their illness.

    b. Causes. The origin of myocarditis remains idiopathic in most cases. *Toxoplasmosis gondii* is the most common AIDS-related opportunistic infection that causes myocarditis.

  2. Cardiomyopathy

    a. Incidence. Dilated cardiomyopathy may occur in as many as 15% of patients with AIDS.

    b. Causes. In patients with AIDS, cardiomyopathy may result from:

      (1) Myocarditis with myocardial fibrosis

      (2) HIV-1 itself

      (3) Cardiotoxic medications (e.g., zidovudine, doxorubicin, interleukin-2, α interferon)

      (4) Cardiotoxicity from nontherapeutic drugs (e.g., ethanol, cocaine, heroin)

HOT KEY Early diagnosis, aggressive treatment, and improved supportive care result in longer survival rates for patients with AIDS; therefore, cardiac complications will likely be encountered more frequently.

V **RHEUMATOLOGIC AND CONNECTIVE TISSUE DISEASES**

A. Systemic lupus erythematosus (SLE) is a rheumatologic disease characterized by the formation of autoantibodies and immune complexes. While SLE can affect nearly all organs, cardiac involvement occurs in roughly 25%–50% of patients.

1. **Pericardial disease.** The pericardium is the most frequent site of cardiovascular disease in patients with SLE.

   a. **Pericarditis** is common. Many cases can be treated with nonsteroidal anti-inflammatory drugs (NSAIDs), but refractory cases may require corticosteroids (e.g, prednisone).

   b. **Pericardial effusion** may also occur. Typically, the pericardial fluid has the following characteristics in patients with SLE:

      (1) An elevated leukocyte count with polymorphonuclear cell predominance

      (2) Acid fluid (i.e., pH < 7)

      (3) An elevated protein concentration

      (4) Low complement levels

      (5) The presence of autoantibodies (e.g., antinuclear or anti-double-stranded DNA antibodies)

2. **Myocardial disease.** Myocarditis and cardiomyopathy are rare, affecting fewer than 10% of patients with SLE.

3. **Valvular disease**

   a. Classically, valvular abnormalities in patients with SLE involve noninfective vegetations (i.e., **marantic** or **Libman-Sacks endocarditis**). Mitral involvement is most common, although SLE can affect any valve.

   b. Complications include valve regurgitation and stenosis, infective endocarditis, and thromboembolism.

   c. Fewer than 10% of patients with SLE will require valve replacement.

4. **CAD**

   a. SLE increases the risk of premature coronary atherosclerosis, particularly when antiphospholipid antibodies are present.

   b. Coronary arteritis can occur. Treatment involves antiplatelet and corticosteroid therapy.

B. Polyarteritis nodosa (PAN) is characterized by necrotizing inflammation affecting the medium- to small-sized arteries throughout the body. The heart frequently is involved, as PAN typically affects the smaller epicardial coronary arteries that penetrate into the myocardium.

1. **Coronary artery vasculitis** may cause thrombi or aneurysms to develop in the coronary arteries, occasionally leading to MI. Glucocorticoid therapy is often used to treat the underlying vasculitis.

    2. Perivascular inflammation of the small arteries of the conduction system may affect the sinoatrial (SA) and atrioventricular (AV) nodes. Patients may develop sick sinus syndrome or AV block.

    3. Systemic hypertension occurs in as many as 90% of patients with PAN, usually accompanied by PAN-related renal dysfunction.

C. Polymyositis and dermatomyositis are idiopathic autoimmune inflammatory myopathies usually accompanied by an elevated serum creatine kinase (CK). Nearly 50% of patients have cardiac abnormalities, including AV block, tachyarrhythmias, pericarditis, coronary artery vasculitis, and dilated cardiomyopathy.

D. Churg-Strauss vasculitis (i.e., allergic granulomatous angiitis), a systemic vasculitis, is accompanied by allergic rhinitis, asthma, and eosinophilia. Dilated cardiomyopathy and mitral regurgitation may occur and account for high morbidity and mortality.

E. Rheumatoid arthritis refers to deforming joint erosion that results from chronic synovial tissue inflammation and proliferation.

    1. Pericardial disease. Acute pericarditis and pericardial effusion may occur. Constrictive pericarditis is rare.

    2. Myocardial disease. Rheumatoid nodules may infiltrate the myocardium in as many as 25% of patients with rheumatoid arthritis. A fraction of these patients may have severe involvement leading to CHF.

    3. Valvular disease. In 1%–2% of patients, rheumatoid nodules may develop within the valve leaflets, leading to valvular regurgitation.

F. Scleroderma (i.e., systemic sclerosis) is a connective tissue disorder characterized by fibrous thickening of the skin and fibrosis of the tissues of the esophagus, intestines, kidneys, lung, and heart. Cardiac involvement is clinically evident in as many as 40% of patients and is an important determinant of mortality.

    1. Pericarditis and **pericardial effusion** may be present in about 20% of patients with scleroderma and is usually attributable to concomitant renal failure.

    2. Diastolic and systolic left ventricular dysfunction may result from patchy myocardial fibrosis and necrosis. Complications include heart failure, MI, arrhythmias, and sudden death.

    3. CAD may result from fibrosis of the epicardial and small coronary arteries. Coronary artery narrowing and occlusion may be present.

G. Ankylosing spondylitis is characterized by progressive inflammation of the spine, leading to chronic back pain, spine immobilization, and deformity. Cardiovascular involvement is generally limited to inflammation of the aortic root; roughly 5% of patients with ankylosing spondylitis experience aortic regurgitation.

H. Marfan's syndrome is associated with defects in the fibrillin-1 gene, resulting in a constellation of clinical features affecting the skeletal, ocular, and cardiovascular systems.

   1. Aortic regurgitation and **ascending aortic root rupture,** which are caused by chronic aortic root dilatation, result in major cardiovascular complications (e.g., CHF, aortic dissection). β Blocker therapy may reduce the patient's risk of aortic root dilatation and rupture.

   2. Mitral valve prolapse (MVP) is common. In severe cases with associated mitral regurgitation, patients may require mitral valve replacement.

   3. Infective endocarditis may also occur in patients with MVP and mitral regurgitation; therefore, antibiotic prophylaxis is recommended (see Chapter 22 VIII C).

VI RENAL DISEASES

A. Pericardial disease

   1. Uremic pericarditis may develop in patients with acute or chronic renal failure. The pathogenesis of this condition remains unclear. The treatment of choice is dialysis.

   2. Pericardial effusions may decrease after dialysis.

   3. Tamponade. Pericardiocentesis may be required for patients with tamponade.

B. Hypertension is commonly seen in patients with acute or chronic renal failure.

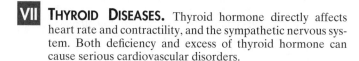

> **HOT** Patients with renal failure may also develop hyperkalemia,
> ▶ which is a serious electrolyte disorder. Complications may in-
>   clude electrocardiographic abnormalities, ventricular arrhyth-
> **KEY** mias, and death from pulseless electrical activity (PEA).

VII THYROID DISEASES.

Thyroid hormone directly affects heart rate and contractility, and the sympathetic nervous system. Both deficiency and excess of thyroid hormone can cause serious cardiovascular disorders.

A. Hypothyroidism (i.e., **myxedema**) results from decreased production of thyroid hormone.

   1. Arrhythmias. Hypothyroidism usually results in sinus bradycardia.

   2. CHF. Hypothyroidism results in reduced cardiac output (CO) and increased peripheral vascular resistance. This frequently results in a narrow pulse pressure and diastolic hypertension. With severe myxedema, ventricular dysfunction and dilatation may occur. Longstanding hypothyroidism can cause CHF.

3. **CAD.** Hypothyroidism is associated with hypercholesterolemia, placing patients at an increased risk for developing CAD. Because of the slow heart rate, however, angina is uncommon unless severe atherosclerotic disease is present.

HOT KEY Thyroid hormone replacement may precipitate CHF and angina, particularly when preexisting myocardial or coronary disease is present. In hypothyroid outpatients with CHF or CAD, start thyroid hormone replacement at low doses (e.g., a 25-μg oral dose of thyroxine daily).

B. **Hyperthyroidism** (i.e., **thyrotoxicosis**) results from chronically elevated levels of thyroid hormone.
   1. **Arrhythmias**
      a. Hyperthyroidism usually results in sinus tachycardia.
      b. Atrial fibrillation may also develop (in roughly 10%–25% of patients) and is particularly common in the elderly.
   2. **CHF** may develop in patients with underlying cardiac disease. Hyperthyroidism often results in increased CO, peripheral vasodilation, systolic hypertension, and diastolic hypotension (i.e., a wide pulse pressure).
   3. **Thromboembolic disease** may occur in patients with hyperthyroidism. In patients with accompanying atrial fibrillation, CHF, and mitral valve disease, the risk of cerebral emboli increases to as much as 40%.

HOT KEY Anticoagulation therapy is important in patients with hyperthyroidism and atrial fibrillation to reduce the risk of thromboembolic disease.

VIII NEOPLASTIC DISEASES

A. **Primary cardiac tumors** are less common than secondary (metastatic) cardiac tumors. Primary tumors usually present as intracavitary masses, and 75% are benign.
   1. **Benign primary tumors**
      a. **Cardiac myxomas** are the most common benign tumors of the heart.
         (1) **Location.** Myxomas are usually attached to the endocardium. Most are located in the left atrium (75%),

but others can also be found in the right atrium
(15%), right ventricle (5%), and left ventricle (5%).

(2) Size. These friable tumors vary from 1–15 cm in diameter.

(3) History. Most patients with a cardiac myxoma present
with the following signs and symptoms.

  (a) Constitutional symptoms (i.e., weight loss, fatigue, fever) are present in 90% of patients.

  (b) Embolization to the brain, kidneys, coronary arteries, or extremities may occur in as many as
  50% of patients. Patients may present with symptoms of weakness or numbness (cerebral embolization), chest pain (coronary embolization),
  or cold or painful extremities (peripheral embolization).

  (c) Obstructive manifestations include syncope (resulting from obstructed blood flow and subsequently reduced CO) and pedal edema (if a right
  atrial tumor obstructs flow from the inferior vena
  cava).

(4) Physical examination

  (a) Heart sounds. A low-frequency **"tumor plop"** is
  best heard at the apex shortly after the second
  heart sound (S_2). This sound is sometimes con-
  fused with an early third heart sound (S_3) or an
  opening snap.

  (b) Murmurs. An apical systolic murmur, diastolic
  murmur, or both may be heard.

(5) Imaging studies. Echocardiography is the most useful
test to localize the cardiac tumor. Computed tomography (CT) or magnetic resonance imaging (MRI)
may be helpful if the echocardiogram is not definitive.

(6) Treatment. Although most myxomas are benign,
complete surgical removal of the tumor is usually recommended to prevent complications resulting from
embolism or obstruction.

  b. Rare benign cardiac neoplasms include rhabdomyoma, fi-
  broma, lipoma, and mesothelioma.

  2. Malignant primary tumors of the heart include angiosar-
  coma, rhabdomyosarcoma, fibrosarcoma, liposarcoma, and
  primary malignant lymphoma.

B. Secondary (metastatic) cardiac tumors involving the heart occur 20–40 times more frequently than primary cardiac tumors.

  1. Location. Secondary tumors are most commonly located in
  the pericardium, resulting in pericarditis or malignant pericardial effusion. Tumors may also be found in the myocardium, endocardium, valves, and coronary arteries.

2. Causes

a. **Direct or lymphatic spread** from lung or breast cancer is the most common cause of cardiac metastases.

b. **Hematogenous spread** accounts for cardiac metastases from malignant melanoma, lymphoma, and leukemia.

HOT **KEY**

Myocardial spread occurs in up to 50% of metastatic melanoma cases.

C. **Carcinoid syndrome** involves tumors, usually found in the gastrointestinal tract, that contain high concentrations of 5-hydroxytryptamine (5-HT). These tumors may cause cutaneous flushing, diarrhea, wheezing, and cardiac lesions.

1. Circulating carcinoids (e.g., serotonin, 5-HT, bradykinin) may lead to the formation of glistening, yellow-white, plaque-like deposits on the tricuspid and pulmonic valves.

2. Contraction caused by these deposits can lead to tricuspid and pulmonic valve regurgitation and right-sided CHF.

References

Hall RJ, Cooley DA, McAllister HA, Frazier OH: Neoplastic heart disease. In *Hurst's The Heart,* 9th ed. Edited by Alexander RW, Schlant RC, Fuster V. New York, McGraw-Hill, 1998, pp 2295–2318.

Michaels AD, Lederman RJ, MacGregor JS, et al: Cardiovascular involvement in AIDS. *Curr Probl Cardiol* 22(3):109–148, 1997.

Moder KG, Miller TD, Tazelaar HD: Cardiac involvement in systemic lupus erythematosus. *Mayo Clin Proc* 74(3):275–284, 1999.

Schenker S, Bay MK: Medical problems associated with alcoholism. *Adv Intern Med* 43:27–78, 1998.

Schlant RC, Gonzalez EB, Roberts WC: The connective tissue diseases. In *Hurst's The Heart,* 9th ed. Edited by Alexander RW, Schlant RC, Fuster V. New York, McGraw-Hill, 1998, pp 2271–2294.

27. Cardiovascular Drug Interactions

I INTRODUCTION

A. **Overview.** Possible drug-drug, drug-food, and drug-herb interactions should be reviewed whenever drug therapy is begun or ended or dosages are adjusted.
   1. Many cardiovascular drugs have important interactions with other drugs, foods, and herbs.
   2. Noncardiovascular drugs also may have important interactions with other drugs, foods, and herbs, which may affect the cardiovascular system.

B. **Definitions**
   1. **Pharmacodynamic interactions** occur when the therapeutic or toxic effects of one drug are altered by another drug.
   2. **Pharmacokinetic interactions** involve the effects of one drug's absorption, protein binding, metabolism, or excretion on another drug.

II INTERACTIONS BETWEEN CARDIOVASCULAR DRUGS

A. **Antihypertensive agents**
   1. **β Blockers**
      a. **Pharmacodynamic interactions**
         (1) When β blockers are combined with verapamil, diltiazem, or digoxin, bradycardia or atrioventricular (AV) block may occur.
         (2) In patients with left ventricular systolic dysfunction, combining β blockers with verapamil or diltiazem may precipitate congestive heart failure (CHF).
         (3) Combining β blockers with other antihypertensive agents may cause hypotension.
      b. **Pharmacokinetic interactions**
         (1) Cigarette smoking and alcohol use increase the cytochrome P-450 system in the liver, thereby reducing the circulating levels of metoprolol, propranolol, and labetolol. Cimetidine and verapamil may reduce the hepatic metabolic rate, leading to increased levels of these β blockers.
         (2) Atenolol, on the other hand, is excreted unchanged in the kidney and is not affected by changes in the hepatic metabolic rate.

226

2. Calcium channel blockers
  a. Pharmacodynamic interactions
     (1) When verapamil or diltiazem is combined with β block-ers or digoxin, bradycardia or AV block may occur.
     (2) In patients with systolic dysfunction, combining verapamil or diltiazem with β blockers may precipi-tate CHF. Amlodipine seems to be a safer calcium blocker for patients with a reduced ejection fraction.
     (3) Combining calcium antagonists with other antihyper-tensive medications may lead to hypotension.
  b. Pharmacokinetic interactions
     (1) Verapamil may inhibit the hepatic oxidation of some drugs, leading to increased levels of prazosin, quinidine, and theophylline. Verapamil may also in-crease digoxin levels by inhibiting digoxin's renal clearance.
     (2) Diltiazem may raise cyclosporine levels by inhibiting cyclosporine's hepatic metabolism.
     (3) Nifedipine may decrease quinidine levels by aug-menting quinidine's hepatic metabolism.
     (4) Cimetidine may lead to increased levels of verapamil, diltiazem, and nifedipine by inhibiting their hepatic metabolism.
3. Nitrates. Excessive hypotension may occur when nitrates are combined with other antihypertensive agents.

HOT KEY For patients receiving any form of nitrate therapy, sildenafil (Vi-agra) should not be prescribed because of the risk of poten-tially life-threatening hypotension.

---

4. Diuretics may have the following pharmacodynamic inter-actions:
  a. Hypokalemia due to diuretics may exacerbate digoxin toxicity. Hypokalemia may also predispose a patient to ventricular arrhythmias, particularly when diuretics are combined with agents that prolong the QT interval (e.g., procainamide, propafenone, flecainide, sotalol, amio-darone, phenothiazines, tricyclic antidepressants).
  b. Captopril may decrease the diuretic effect of furosemide.
  c. Estrogens and nonsteroidal anti-inflammatory drugs (NSAIDs) may decrease the antihypertensive effect of thiazide diuretics.
5. Angiotensin-converting enzyme (ACE) inhibitors
  a. Pharmacodynamic interactions
     (1) Potassium-sparing diuretics (e.g., spironolactone) or

potassium supplements combined with ACE inhibitors can lead to hyperkalemia.

(2) Aspirin and NSAIDs can attenuate the vasodilatory effects of ACE inhibitors, possibly diminishing the benefits of ACE inhibitors in patients with heart failure.

b. Pharmacokinetic interactions. Captopril may decrease the renal clearance of digoxin by roughly 20%–30%.

B. Antiarrhythmics

1. Quinidine

a. Pharmacodynamic interactions

(1) Drugs that cause hypokalemia (e.g., diuretics) may decrease the antiarrhythmic effects of quinidine and may increase the risk of ventricular tachyarrhythmias by prolonging the QT interval.

(2) When quinidine is combined with another drug that prolongs the QT interval, the risk of ventricular arrhythmias may increase.

b. Pharmacokinetic interactions. Quinidine significantly increases the levels of digoxin and warfarin. Therefore, doses of digoxin and warfarin may need to be reduced by roughly 50% in patients who are taking quinidine (Table 27-1).

2. Amiodarone

a. Pharmacodynamic interactions

(1) When amiodarone is combined with β blockers, verapamil, or diltiazem, excessive bradycardia may occur.

(2) When amiodarone is combined with another agent that prolongs the QT interval, the risk of torsades de pointes may increase.

b. Pharmacokinetic interactions. Amiodarone significantly increases the levels of digoxin and warfarin. Therefore, doses of digoxin and warfarin usually need to be reduced by roughly 50% in patients who are taking amiodarone (see Table 27-1).

HOT

KEY

Because of amiodarone's long half-life, drug interactions may persist for several weeks after amiodarone has been stopped.

C. Digoxin

1. Pharmacodynamic interactions

a. Diuretics may cause hypokalemia, which can then precipitate digoxin toxicity.

TABLE 27-1. Pharmacokinetic Interactions Associated with Warfarin

Interaction Effect	Drug Class	Drugs
Increased PT	Cardiac	Amiodarone, propafenone, quinidine, propranolol, gemfibrozil, lovastatin, simvastatin
	Antibiotic	Cotrimoxazole, erythromycin, fluconazole, isoniazid, itraconazole, metronidazole, miconazole
	Anti-inflammatory	Allopurinol, piroxicam
	Gastrointestinal	Cimetidine, omeprazole
Decreased PT	Cardiac	Cholestyramine, colestipol
	Antibiotic	Griseofulvin, nafcillin, rifampin
	Central nervous	Barbiturates, carbamazepine, chlordiazepoxide
	Gastrointestinal	Sucralfate
	Dietary	Substances high in vitamin K (e.g., vitamin K supplements, broccoli, avocado)

PT = prothrombin time.

  b. When digoxin is combined with β blockers, verapamil, or diltiazem, AV block may occur.
 2. Pharmacokinetic interactions
  a. Verapamil increases digoxin levels by 60%–90%. Nifedipine and diltiazem also increase digoxin levels, but not quite as much as verapamil.
  b. Quinidine, propafenone, and amiodarone roughly double digoxin levels in the blood.
  c. Cholestyramine may impair digoxin absorption.
D. Hypolipidemics
 1. Statins (e.g., HMG CoA reductase inhibitors) are generally well tolerated but have the potential for important drug interactions.
  a. Pharmacodynamic interactions
   (1) The use of a statin in combination with gemfibrozil,

cyclosporine, or erythromycin increases the risk of myopathy and rhabdomyolysis.

(2) The use of niacin with a statin may increase this risk slightly but is considered a relatively safe combination.

b. **Pharmacokinetic interactions.** Lovastatin and simvastatin may slightly increase the prothrombin time in patients taking warfarin (see Table 27-1).

2. **Niacin** (nicotinic acid) may have the following pharmacodynamic interactions:

a. When combined with clonidine, niacin may exacerbate orthostatic hypotension.

b. Niacin may increase serum glucose levels, requiring adjustment of hypoglycemic medications in patients with diabetes.

c. Niacin may increase uric acid levels, requiring adjustment of hypouricemic medications in patients with gout.

3. **Fibrates** (e.g., gemfibrozil)

a. **Pharmacodynamic interactions.** The use of a fibrate in combination with a statin significantly increases the risk of myopathy and rhabdomyolysis. These risks are particularly increased for patients with hepatic or renal insufficiency, known myopathy, and those taking immunosuppressive agents.

b. **Pharmacokinetic interactions.** Gemfibrozil may increase the prothrombin time in patients taking warfarin (see Table 27-1).

4. **Resin** (bile acid-binders). Most drug interactions with resin agents are pharmacokinetic and are related to impaired absorption of other medications (e.g., β blockers, amiodarone, thiazide diuretics, thyroid hormone, warfarin). Therefore, it is recommended that patients take other medications at least 1 hour before or 4 hours after taking the resin. Patients should take resins with meals.

E. **Antithrombotic agents**

1. **Aspirin** may have the following pharmacodynamic interactions:

a. Aspirin combined with other antiplatelet agents or warfarin may increase the risk of bleeding complications.

b. Aspirin may decrease the vasodilatory effects of ACE inhibitors, potentially diminishing their benefits in patients with heart failure.

c. Aspirin reduces the diuretic effects of spironolactone.

2. **Warfarin**

a. **Pharmacodynamic interactions.** Warfarin combined with antiplatelet agents (e.g., aspirin, ticlopidine, clopidogrel) may increase the risk of bleeding complications.

b. **Pharmacokinetic interactions** with warfarin are common and potentially dangerous (see Table 27-1).

III INTERACTIONS BETWEEN NONCARDIOVASCULAR DRUGS may affect the cardiovascular system.

A. Nonsedating antihistamines
1. Terfenadine (Seldane) and astemizole (Hismanal) can prolong cardiac repolarization, leading to QT interval prolongation and torsades de pointes. These medications have been removed from the United States market. The risk for arrhythmia is increased in patients:
   a. Taking other medications that may prolong the QT interval (e.g., erythromycin, clarithromycin, ketoconazole, itraconazole, cisapride, protease inhibitors)
   b. With preexisting QT interval prolongation
   c. With hepatic dysfunction
2. Loratadine (Claritin), cetirizine (Zyrtec), and fexofenadine (Allegra) do not seem to prolong the QT interval or induce ventricular tachyarrhythmias.

B. Antipsychotics and **tricyclic antidepressants** may cause electrocardiographic changes (e.g., QRS and QT prolongation) and serious ventricular arrhythmias. Cardiotoxicity may result from an overdose or when these agents are combined with other medications that prolong the QT interval.
1. Of the neuroleptics, the phenothiazine thioridazine is associated with the highest risk of arrhythmia when used with other medications that prolong the QT interval.
2. Selective serotonin reuptake inhibitors (e.g., fluoxetine, paroxetine, sertraline) have a lower incidence of cardiac complications compared to tricyclic antidepressants (e.g., amitriptyline, nortriptyline, desipramine).

IV INTERACTIONS BETWEEN CARDIOVASCULAR DRUGS AND HERBAL MEDICATIONS.

Roughly 60 million Americans each year use herbal medications. More than two-thirds of these patients do not reveal to their health care providers that they have used herbs. Important cardiovascular drug-herb interactions include the following:

A. Digoxin may have interactions with the following:
1. Herbs (e.g., uzara root, hawthorn, adonis, milkweed, and lily of the valley) that contain digoxin-like substances may lead to digoxin toxicity in patients taking digoxin.
2. Plantain (which is used as an herbal laxative) because it has been reported to have been adulterated with foxglove and can therefore lead to increased digoxin levels in patients taking digoxin.
3. St. John's wort, an herbal antidepressant, decreases digoxin levels by 30%.

HOT KEY Siberian ginseng and kyushin may interfere with digoxin assays, leading to spuriously elevated digoxin levels without true digoxin toxicity.

B. Diuretics
   1. Pharmacodynamic interactions
      a. Sodium-sparing herbal aquaretics (e.g., goldenseal, dandelion, uva ursi) may antagonize the antihypertensive effects of diuretics.
      b. Licorice (which herbalists have used as an antispasmodic herb in peptic ulcer disease) may offset the effects of spironolactone. Licorice can also lead to sodium retention, hypertension, and hypokalemia.
   2. Pharmacokinetic interactions. Gossypol (which herbalists have used for birth control) may lead to increased urinary secretion of potassium, potentially causing hypokalemia. Combining gossypol with other diuretics and digoxin may increase the risk for digoxin toxicity.
C. Warfarin may have pharmacokinetic interactions with the following:
   1. Garlic, ginger, ginkgo, chamomile, and feverfew may increase the effect of warfarin, possibly increasing the risk for hemorrhage.
   2. Ginseng may decrease the effect of warfarin.

HOT KEY St. John's wort acts as an inducer of the hepatic enzyme cytochrome P-450 3A4, leading to increased metabolism of agents such as amiodarone, lidocaine, propafenone, nifedipine, diltiazem, verapamil, amlodipine, felodipine, atorvastatin, cerivastatin, lovastatin, and simvastatin.

References
Bays HE, Duovne CA: Drug interactions of lipid-altering drugs. *Drug Saf* 19:355–371, 1998.
Blaufarb I, Pfeifer TM, Frishman WH: Beta-blockers: drug interactions of clinical significance. *Drug Saf* 13:359–370, 1995.
Cheitlin MD, Hutter AM, Brindis RG, et al: Use of sildenafil (Viagra) in patients with cardiovascular disease. American College of Cardiology/American Heart Association Expert Consensus Document. *J Am Coll Cardiol* 33:273–382, 1999.
Gonzalez MA, Estes KS: Pharmacokinetic overview of oral second-generation H1 antihistamines. *Int J Clin Pharmacol Ther* 36:292–300, 1998.
Jafari-Fesharaki M, Scheinman MM: Adverse effects of amiodarone. *Pacing Clin Electrophysiol* 21:108–120, 1998.
Magnani B, Malini PL: Cardiac glycosides: drug interactions of clinical significance. *Drug Saf* 12:97–109, 1995.

Miller LG: Herbal medicinals: selected clinical considerations focusing on known or
    potential drug-herb interactions. *Arch Intern Med* 158:2200–2211, 1998.
Opie LH: Adverse cardiovascular drug interactions. In *Hurst's the Heart,* 9th ed. Edited
    by Alexander RW, Schlant RC, Fuster V. New York, McGraw-Hill, pp 2371–2388,
    1998.

PART IX

SPECIAL SITUATIONS

28. Pregnancy

I **INTRODUCTION.** A systematic approach to managing and treating a pregnant patient with cardiovascular disease is important.

A. **Heart disease** in a pregnant woman may pose a serious threat to both the mother and fetus.
B. **Many cardiac medications** may be harmful to the fetus; therefore, the use of cardiac medications during pregnancy must be chosen carefully.

II **APPROACH TO THE PREGNANT PATIENT**

A. **History** should focus on symptoms, prior history of cardiac disease, prior pregnancies, and family history of heart disease.
   1. **Symptoms**
      a. Some symptoms of heart disease (e.g., fatigue, dyspnea, chest pain, palpitations, and lightheadedness) are also common complaints in normal pregnancy.
      b. Severe dyspnea that limits daily activities, hemoptysis, and exertional syncope are significant findings that warrant closer evaluation.
   2. **Prior history of cardiac disease.** Determine whether the patient has any history of rheumatic heart disease, cardiomyopathy, or hypertension.
   3. **Prior pregnancies**
      a. Ask if maternal hypertension occurred during a prior pregnancy.
      b. Determine if there is a history of congenital heart disease in any prior children.
   4. **Family history of heart disease.** A family history of congenital heart disease or cardiomyopathy may increase the risk of heart disease in the pregnant patient or the fetus.
B. **Physical examination.** The physician should check for signs of valvular or myocardial dysfunction.
   1. Keep in mind that peripheral edema, visible neck pulsations,

a diffuse apical impulse, a third heart sound (S_3), and systolic murmurs are not uncommon findings in a normal pregnancy.

2. Cyanosis, a grade 3/6 systolic murmur or higher, and any diastolic murmur are not normal and should prompt further evaluation.

C. Diagnostic studies

1. **12-Lead electrocardiogram (ECG).** Nonspecific ST/T wave abnormalities have been reported in normal pregnancy. Signs of ventricular hypertrophy or bundle branch block should prompt further evaluation.

2. **Echocardiogram.** A cardiac echocardiogram is safe and can be used to assess the structure and function of the maternal and fetal hearts. The test is particularly useful in patients with preexisting cardiomyopathy, valvular disease, or Marfan's syndrome.

HOT KEY

Radiography, radionuclide studies, and cardiac catheterization requiring fluoroscopy should generally be avoided, particularly early in pregnancy, because of their increased risk of causing infant leukemia and organ maldevelopment.

III NORMAL CARDIOVASCULAR CHANGES IN PREGNANCY.

Significant hemodynamic adjustments occur during pregnancy that can severely affect cardiac function in a pregnant woman with preexisting cardiac disease.

A. Sodium and water retention occur normally during pregnancy.

1. **Total body water** increases steadily during pregnancy by 6–8 L.

2. **Total body sodium** increases by 500–900 meq.

B. Resting cardiac output (CO) increases by 30%–50% by the second trimester and remains elevated throughout the duration of the pregnancy.

1. Increased heart rate and stroke volume result in increased CO and decreased vascular resistance.

2. With each contraction during labor, CO increases up to 50%, and oxygen consumption increases up to 150%.

IV CARDIOVASCULAR DISEASE IN PREGNANCY

A. Maternal congenital heart disease is the most common cause of maternal heart disease in the United States.

1. **High-risk conditions**

a. **Prognosis.** High-risk conditions are associated with high rates of maternal and fetal complications. If severe symptoms develop during pregnancy, the maternal and fetal mortality rates are roughly 30% and 7% respectively. The most common causes of high-risk conditions affecting patients during pregnancy include:

(1) Severe pulmonary hypertension (i.e., primary or secondary), which is associated with a nearly 50% maternal and perinatal mortality

(2) Eisenmenger's syndrome (i.e., severe pulmonary hypertension with a resulting right-to-left shunt), which is associated with a 50%–70% maternal and perinatal mortality

(3) Cyanotic congenital heart disease (i.e., right-to-left intracardiac shunt)

(4) Moderate to severe valvular stenosis

(5) Severe valvular insufficiency

(6) Coarctation of the aorta

b. Treatment. Many of these conditions, particularly severe pulmonary hypertension and Eisenmenger's syndrome, are considered contraindications to pregnancy.

(1) Preconception counseling should be considered for women at high risk for maternal and fetal complications. If the risk is significantly high, **sterilization** or **therapeutic abortion** should be considered.

(2) Hospitalization, with bedrest and close hemodynamic monitoring, is necessary if the fetus is carried to term.

(3) Endocarditis prophylaxis is generally recommended during delivery (see Chapter 22).

2. Low-risk conditions

a. Prognosis. Low-risk conditions generally do not pose a threat during pregnancy, and most asymptomatic patients do well. Common cardiac abnormalities in this group include:

(1) Atrial septal defect (ASD), ventricular septal defect (VSD), or **patent ductus arteriosus (PDA)** with normal pulmonary artery pressures

(2) Mild to moderate valvular stenosis or **insufficiency**

b. Treatment. Patients generally need close follow-up and monitoring for the development of symptoms and complications during pregnancy.

B. Valvular disease

HOT KEY

Rheumatic heart disease is the most common cause of maternal heart disease worldwide and the second most common cause in the United States.

1. **Mitral stenosis**
   a. **Incidence.** Mitral stenosis is the most common valvular complication of rheumatic heart disease found in women of childbearing age.
   b. **Prognosis.** Symptoms (e.g., dyspnea, hemoptysis) usually develop in roughly 25% of patients with severe mitral stenosis by the twentieth week of pregnancy as a result of pulmonary vascular congestion. Labor may further exacerbate symptoms.
   c. **Treatment**
      (1) **Mitral balloon valvuloplasty** (with appropriate radiation shielding to protect the fetus) is the treatment of choice for pregnant women with symptomatic mitral stenosis.
      (2) **Endocarditis prophylaxis** is recommended for women with a complicated vaginal delivery (see Chapter 22).
      (3) Daily **digoxin** therapy may be considered to reduce the risk of rapid ventricular response in patients with atrial fibrillation.
      (4) **Anticoagulation therapy** is indicated for patients with atrial fibrillation.
2. **Aortic valve disorders** (e.g., congenital bicuspid aortic valve, aortic stenosis) are rare in women of childbearing age.
3. **Prosthetic heart valves**
   a. **Incidence.** During pregnancy, the risks associated with prosthetic heart valves (i.e., thromboemboli, bleeding, and endocarditis) increase. Complications occur in approximately 2%–4% of women.
   b. **Treatment**
      (1) **Anticoagulation** is essential during pregnancy for women with mechanical heart valves.
         (a) Warfarin is contraindicated in the first trimester. For women considering pregnancy, warfarin should be stopped prior to conception and substituted with **subcutaneous heparin** (usually 10,000–15,000 units twice daily) to keep the partial thromboplastin time 1.5–2.0 times normal. Low-molecular-weight heparin (e.g., enoxaparin; 1 mg/kg subcutaneously twice daily) may be a good alternative to standard heparin.
         (b) In the second and third trimesters, patients may switch back to warfarin. If warfarin is used, however, patients must switch back to heparin from 35–37 weeks until delivery.
         (c) When labor begins, heparin should be stopped and restarted 2–4 hours postpartum.

      (d) Warfarin can be restarted 1 day after delivery because it does not enter the breast milk.

    (2) Endocarditis prophylaxis is recommended (see Chapter 22).

  4. Infectious endocarditis is a serious infection, which may occur during pregnancy.

    a. Prevention is always important during pregnancy. Antibiotic prophylaxis should be used in high-risk patients undergoing dental or surgical procedures (see Chapter 22).

    b. Treatment involves consultation with an infectious disease specialist and includes intravenous antibiotics.

C. Hypertension may either improve or worsen during pregnancy.

  1. Preexisting hypertension. Chances of fetal mortality are only slightly higher than normal when preexisting hypertension is controlled.

    a. Nonpharmacologic therapy includes bedrest and a low sodium diet. In order to reduce the risks associated with cardiac medications, patients with a blood pressure of 160/100 mm Hg or lower may be treated nonpharmacologically during pregnancy.

    b. Pharmacologic therapy. For patients with a blood pressure higher than 160/100 mm Hg, antihypertensive therapy should be continued during pregnancy. Angiotensin-converting enzyme (ACE) inhibitors, thiazide diuretics, spironolactone, and reserpine should be stopped and substituted with safer alternatives. (Tables 28-1 and 28-2 a list of drugs that are generally safe and unsafe during pregnancy.)

  2. Gestational hypertension is defined as asymptomatic systemic hypertension that begins during pregnancy.

    a. Nonpharmacologic therapy includes bedrest and a low sodium diet.

    b. Pharmacologic therapy is indicated when the patient's systolic blood pressure is greater than or equal to 160 mm Hg or diastolic blood pressure is greater than or equal to 100 mm Hg (see Tables 28-1 and 28-2).

      (1) The drug of choice is **methyldopa** (250–1000 mg orally three times daily).

      (2) Hydralazine, β blockers, α blockers, or calcium channel blockers may be added if necessary.

      (3) Avoid ACE inhibitors, thiazide diuretics, spironolactone, and reserpine.

  3. Preeclampsia should be considered when a woman is hypertensive during the third trimester, particularly if she also has significant proteinuria ($\geq$ 500 mg/dL/day), headache, visual disturbances, or epigastric pain. If the patient also develops convulsions or coma, **eclampsia** is diagnosed and the maternal mortality increases to 10%–15%.

TABLE 28-1. Medications That Are Generally Safe During Pregnancy*	
Medications	**Medical Conditions**
Heparin	Mechanical heart valves
Low-molecular-weight heparin	Deep venous thrombosis
	Hypercoagulable states with prior thromboembolic complications
Lidocaine	Arrhythmias
Quinidine	
Adenosine	Supraventricular tachyarrhythmias
Digoxin	Congestive heart failure
	Atrial fibrillation
Methyldopa	Hypertension
Hydralazine	
Nitrates	
β Blockers (e.g., metoprolol, labetalol)	
α Blockers (e.g., prazosin, terazosin)	
Calcium channel blockers (e.g., nifedipine, diltiazem, verapamil)	
Furosemide	Congestive heart failure
Dobutamine	

*These medications do not appear to be associated with significant complications for the fetus; however, adequate studies concerning medication safety are lacking.

    a. Nonpharmacologic therapy includes hospitalization and bedrest for moderate and severe cases.

    b. Pharmacologic therapy is paramount to maintain the diastolic blood pressure at or below 95 mm Hg and the mean blood pressure at 100–110 mm Hg. Intravenous **hydralazine** and **labetalol** are useful agents.

    c. Delivery is indicated for uncontrolled hypertension, progressive renal insufficiency or liver dysfunction, and signs of eclampsia.

D. Myocardial disease

  1. Preexisting congestive heart failure (CHF)

    a. Prognosis. Preexisting CHF places the mother and fetus at increased risk if congestive symptoms (e.g., dyspnea) occur with minimal exertion. Women with severe cardiomyopathy should generally avoid pregnancy.

    b. Treatment. Preexisting CHF should be treated with stan-

TABLE 28-2. Medications That Are Generally Unsafe During Pregnancy*

Medications	Possible Risk
Warfarin†	May cause severe organ malformations in 15%–25% of fetuses exposed during the first 2 months May cause hemorrhage if taken late in pregnancy
Aspirin	May increase the risk of abortion and fetal growth retardation
Indomethacin	May cause closure of the ductus arteriosus during fetal life by inhibiting prostaglandin synthesis
ACE inhibitors Angiotensin receptor antagonists	May affect renal function in the fetus
Nitroprusside‡	May result in accumulation of cyanide and thiocyanate in the fetus
Thiazide diuretics Spironolactone Diazoxide Reserpine	May pose significant risk to fetal development

*These medications have been shown to be associated with serious risk to the fetus (by crossing the placental barrier) and should be avoided during pregnancy. ACE = angiotensin-converting enzyme.
†Patients can resume warfarin therapy 1 day after an uncomplicated delivery.
‡Short-term therapy (i.e., < 1–2 days) may be considered in selected patients.

dard therapy (i.e., furosemide, digoxin, hydralazine, and nitrates). Women should avoid ACE inhibitors during pregnancy.

2. Peripartum cardiomyopathy (PPCM)

    a. Incidence. PPCM occurs in roughly 1 out of 10,000 pregnancies, usually between 1 month before and 6 months after delivery.

    b. Prognosis. The natural history varies widely. Some patients recover completely, while others progress to refractory heart failure.

    c. Treatment. Patients with PPCM should be treated for systolic dysfunction. Dobutamine may be added for patients whose conditions are refractory to standard therapy (i.e., furosemide, digoxin, hydralazine, and nitrates).

3. **Hypertrophic cardiomyopathy** often results in increased severity of symptoms during pregnancy.
  a. **Prognosis.** Symptomatic hypertrophic cardiomyopathy places the mother and fetus at increased risk for adverse events.
  b. **Treatment.** Medical therapy for patients with hypertrophic cardiomyopathy is described in Chapter 16 VI D 2 d.
    (1) During pregnancy, women should avoid β-sympathomimetic tocolytic therapy (e.g., terbutaline) and hypovolemia.
    (2) **Endocarditis prophylaxis** is recommended (see Chapter 22).

E. **Aortic dissection**
  1. **Incidence.** Aortic dissection, a rare complication of pregnancy, typically occurs near term or shortly postpartum. Patients with **Marfan's syndrome** are at particularly high risk for aortic dissection; therefore, surveillance echocardiograms should be obtained during pregnancy for patients with Marfan's syndrome.
  2. **Treatment**
    a. **Medical therapy** includes aggressive antihypertensive therapy (e.g., intravenous nitroprusside, labetalol) in the intensive care unit.
    b. **Surgical repair** is reserved for patients with a type-A dissection (i.e., one that involves the ascending aorta).
    c. **Special precautions** should be used for patients with **Marfan's syndrome.**
      (1) **Therapeutic abortion** should be considered for pregnant women with significant aortic root dilatation (> 40–45 mm in diameter) because of the high risk of aortic dissection.
      (2) **β Blockers** and **bedrest** should be considered to reduce the risk of aortic dilatation.
      (3) **Cesarean delivery** is recommended to avoid the hemodynamic stresses of labor.

References

Khedun SM, Moodley J, Naicker T, et al: Drug management of hypertensive disorders of pregnancy. *Pharmacol Ther* 74:221–258, 1997.

McAnulty JH, Metcalfe J, Ueland K: Heart disease and pregnancy. In *Hurst's The Heart,* 9th ed. Edited by Alexander RW, Schlant RC, Fuster V. New York, McGraw-Hill, 1998, pp 2389–2406.

Perloff D: Hypertension and pregnancy-related hypertension. *Cardiol Clin* 16:79–101, 1998.

Sibai BM: Treatment of hypertension in pregnant women. *N Engl J Med* 335:257–265, 1996.

Teerlink JR, Foster E: Valvular heart disease in pregnancy. A contemporary perspective. *Cardiol Clin* 16:573–598, 1998.

29. Geriatric Cardiology

I **INTRODUCTION.** Estimates are that 50 million people in the United States (roughly 1 in 5) are older than 65 years. Coronary artery disease (CAD), arrhythmias, congestive heart failure (CHF), valvular heart disease, and hypertension are more common among patients in this age group. Therefore, it is important for physicians to be able to recognize age-related changes in cardiovascular function and know how to manage an elderly patient with cardiovascular disease.

II **CARDIOVASCULAR CHANGES ASSOCIATED WITH AGING**

A. **Cardiovascular structure**
  1. **Myocardial changes**
     a. The left ventricle becomes hypertrophied.
     b. Myocardial collagen deposition increases.
     c. A progressive, age-associated loss of myocytes occurs in both ventricles as well as in the conduction system [e.g., sinoatrial (SA) node, atrioventricular (AV) node, His bundle].
  2. **Valvular changes**
     a. The aortic and mitral leaflets thicken.
     b. Calcification of the mitral valve (i.e., mitral annular calcification) is common.
  3. **Vasculature changes.** The arterial walls develop increased collagen content, intimal thickness, and elastin fragmentation.
B. **Cardiovascular function.** Changes in cardiovascular function reflect the structural changes discussed in II A.
  1. **Myocardial changes.** The myocardium becomes less compliant, thus impairing diastolic relaxation. Diastolic dysfunction may result (see Chapter 16 II C 2).
  2. **Valvular changes.** Aortic and mitral regurgitation are more common in the elderly than in younger patients.
  3. **Vasculature changes.** Because the arterial vasculature becomes less elastic, the prevalence of hypertension increases.

III **CORONARY ARTERY DISEASE** accounts for 80% of deaths among patients older than 65 years.

A. **Chronic ischemic heart disease** (see Chapter 12). In general, geriatric patients tend to have more severe and extensive CAD compared to younger patients with ischemic heart disease.

1. **Epidemiology**
   a. By age 70, nearly 1 in 6 men and 1 in 10 women have CAD.
   b. By age 80, roughly 1 in 5 men and women have CAD.
   c. By age 90, over one-third of people have at least one coronary artery occlusion.
2. **Causes.** Coronary artery atherosclerosis is the primary cause of CAD.
3. **Treatment** of elderly patients with ischemic heart disease is similar to that recommended for younger patients; however, several issues should be emphasized.
   a. Elderly patients may be more susceptible to drug-induced hypotension and AV block. Therefore, antianginal medications should generally be started at the lowest recommended doses (see Appendix B).
   b. Advanced age alone is not a contraindication to angioplasty and coronary artery bypass graft (CABG) surgery. Because the surgical complication rate is higher for elderly patients, careful patient selection is important before revascularization.

B. **Acute myocardial infarction** (AMI) [see Chapter 13]
   1. **Epidemiology.** The incidence of AMI increases steadily with age. In fact, 50% of patients hospitalized for AMI are older than 65 years. Older patients may be less likely to report early symptoms of AMI (e.g., chest pain) and instead wait until later, more severe symptoms develop (e.g., dyspnea).
   2. **Treatment.** Thrombolysis is effective in restoring coronary blood flow, salvaging ischemic myocardium, and reducing mortality in elderly patients with AMI. While the risk of cerebral hemorrhage increases in elderly patients who receive thrombolytic agents, the overall mortality is greatly reduced.

HOT **KEY**   Aggressive treatment should not be withheld from geriatric patients with AMI. While older patients have higher morbidity and mortality rates from AMI compared to younger patients, they also have the highest expected benefit from proven therapies, such as thrombolytics, aspirin, and β blockers.

IV **ARRHYTHMIAS**

A. **Atrial fibrillation** (see Chapter 8)
   1. **Epidemiology.** Atrial fibrillation is present in 5% of the general population older than 60 years and 10% of the general population older than 80 years.

2. Causes. Atrial fibrillation in elderly patients most commonly results from CAD, hypertension, CHF, or valvular heart disease. "Lone" atrial fibrillation is less common in elderly patients than in younger patients.

3. Treatment. Anticoagulation therapy (with warfarin) is recommended for elderly patients with atrial fibrillation, unless they have a contraindication to anticoagulation (e.g., a high risk for falls).

B. Sinus node dysfunction (i.e., sick sinus syndrome) includes several arrhythmias, such as tachycardia–bradycardia syndrome, sinus bradycardia, sinus pause, or sinus arrest.

1. Epidemiology. Sinus node dysfunction primarily affects the elderly.

2. Causes. The most common cause is idiopathic degeneration of the SA node. Other causes include CAD, prior cardiac surgery, and medications (e.g., β blockers, calcium channel blockers).

3. Treatment. Any medications that slow conduction in the SA node (e.g., β blockers, verapamil, diltiazem, amiodarone, sotalol) should be stopped if possible. Digoxin may help patients with symptomatic supraventricular tachyarrhythmias. Patients may require implantation of a dual-chamber pacemaker.

C. Ventricular arrhythmias are more common in the elderly than in younger patients. Premature ventricular complexes (PVCs) increase in frequency with advancing age. Work-up and management of ventricular tachyarrhythmias are discussed in Chapter 9.

V CONGESTIVE HEART FAILURE

A. Epidemiology

1. CHF is common in older patients, affecting roughly 2 million elderly Americans.

2. Starting after age 50, the prevalence of CHF doubles every 7 years among women and every 10 years among men.

B. Causes

1. Diastolic dysfunction in elderly patients results primarily from CAD and hypertension.

2. Systolic dysfunction, which accounts for nearly 50% of cases of CHF in elderly patients, primarily results from MI, hypertension, and valvular heart disease.

3. Many patients have both diastolic and systolic dysfunction.

C. Treatment. Because treatment for diastolic dysfunction differs from that for systolic dysfunction, assessment of left ventricular systolic function is recommended for patients with CHF (see Chapter 16 IV C–D).

VI **VALVULAR HEART DISEASE.** While the epidemiology and causes of valvular heart disease are different in the elderly, treatment strategies are the same as for younger patients. (Discussion of treatment can be found in Chapters 17 and 18.)

A. **Aortic stenosis** (see Chapter 17)
   1. **Epidemiology.** Aortic stenosis is the most common valvular disorder seen in elderly patients. The prevalence of aortic valve calcific degeneration increases steadily with age.
   2. **Causes.** Senile calcific degeneration is the most common cause of aortic stenosis in elderly patients. Congenital commissural fusion and rheumatic heart disease are much less common causes.
B. **Aortic regurgitation** (see Chapter 17)
   1. **Epidemiology.** While severe aortic regurgitation is less common than aortic stenosis in elderly patients, some degree of aortic regurgitation can be detected in as many as one-third of patients older than 75 years.
   2. **Causes**
      a. Hypertension and aortic root dilatation are the most common causes of chronic aortic regurgitation in elderly patients. Less frequent causes are congenital valve disease, rheumatic fever, and syphilis.
      b. Ascending aortic dissection, endocarditis, or trauma may cause acute aortic regurgitation.
C. **Mitral regurgitation** (see Chapter 18)
   1. **Epidemiology.** Mitral regurgitation is encountered frequently in elderly patients.
   2. **Causes**
      a. In elderly patients, mitral regurgitation most commonly develops as a result of chronic myxomatous degeneration of the mitral valve. Of all patients with mitral valve prolapse (MVP), elderly patients have the highest risk for mitral regurgitation.
      b. Mitral annular calcification, papillary muscle dysfunction related to ischemic heart disease, and hypertensive heart disease are other common causes of mitral regurgitation in this age group.
D. **Mitral stenosis** (see Chapter 18)
   1. **Epidemiology.** Mitral stenosis is rare in elderly patients.
   2. **Causes.** Rheumatic heart disease is the most common cause of mitral stenosis.

VII HYPERTENSION (see Chapter 23)

A. Epidemiology
   1. About two-thirds of Americans older than 65 years have hypertension (i.e., systolic blood pressure > 140 mm Hg or diastolic blood pressure > 90 mm Hg).
   2. Four in ten elderly patients have isolated systolic hypertension (i.e., systolic blood pressure > 140 mm Hg and diastolic blood pressure < 90 mm Hg).

B. Causes
   1. **Essential hypertension** is the most common cause.
   2. **Age-related changes** may lead to an increased prevalence of hypertension in the elderly. These changes include:
      a. Increased salt sensitivity
      b. Renal changes (e.g., decreased renal blood flow, increased renal sodium retention)
      c. Hormonal changes (e.g., increased plasma renin, increased serum norepinephrine and angiotensin II)
      d. Decreased arterial compliance
      e. Decreased α- and β-adrenergic receptor responsiveness
   3. **Renovascular lesions** resulting from atherosclerosis account for most reversible causes of hypertension in the elderly.

C. Treatment of hypertension in elderly patients is similar to that recommended for younger patients. Geriatric patients, however, may have age-related changes that cause pharmacokinetic interactions (see Chapter 27).
   1. **Antihypertensive agents** may need to be administered in lower doses (see Appendix B).
   2. **β Blockers** should be used with caution in elderly patients with conduction disease, CHF, or depression.

HOT **KEY** Diuretics are particularly effective and generally well tolerated by elderly patients with isolated systolic hypertension.

References

Duncan AK, Vittone J, Fleming KC, et al: Cardiovascular disease in elderly patients. *Mayo Clin Proc* 71:184–196, 1996.

Keller NM, Feit F: Coronary artery disease in the geriatric population. *Prog Cardiovasc Dis* 38:407–418, 1996.

Nolan PE, Marcus FI: Geriatric considerations in cardiovascular therapy. In *Hurst's The Heart,* 9th ed. Edited by Alexander RW, Schlant RC, Fuster V. New York, McGraw-Hill, 1998, pp 2451–2457.

Wei JY: Age and the cardiovascular system. *N Engl J Medicine* 327:1735–1739, 1992.

30. Perioperative Evaluation for Noncardiac Surgery

I INTRODUCTION

A. Incidence

1. Of the 25 million Americans who have noncardiac surgery each year, roughly 50,000 will have perioperative myocardial infarction (MI).
2. More than 20,000 deaths following noncardiac surgery result from MI or some other cardiac event, such as unstable angina, congestive heart failure (CHF), or serious arrhythmia.

B. Overview

1. An organized approach should be used to estimate a patient's perioperative risk for an adverse cardiac event.
2. If the patient has a preexisting cardiac disorder, strategies should be implemented to minimize the risk of a perioperative cardiac complication.
3. If cardiac complications do develop postoperatively, they should be carefully managed.

II PREOPERATIVE APPROACH TO THE PATIENT. Preoperative risk assessment involves an evaluation of both the surgical procedure and the patient.

A. Evaluation of the surgical procedure. The term "surgical clearance" should be avoided since every surgical procedure entails some risk. The type of surgery, however, greatly affects the risk for an adverse cardiac event. For example, the risk of postoperative MI or cardiac death increases fourfold when surgery is performed emergently rather than electively.

1. **High-risk procedures** are associated with a cardiovascular risk (i.e., MI, stroke, or death) of 5% or greater. Examples include:
   a. Emergent major operations (e.g., intrathoracic or intraperitoneal trauma surgery)
   b. Major vascular surgery (e.g., abdominal aneurysm repair)
   c. Peripheral vascular surgery (e.g., aortofemoral bypass)
   d. Anticipated prolonged surgery with large fluid shifts or blood loss (e.g., liver transplantation)
2. **Intermediate-risk procedures** are associated with a cardiovascular risk of less than 5% but greater than or equal to 1%. Examples include:

      a. Carotid endarterectomy

      b. Intrathoracic or intraperitoneal surgery

      c. Orthopedic surgery

  3. Low-risk procedures are associated with a cardiovascular risk of less than 1%. Examples include:

      a. Endoscopic procedures

      b. Cataract procedures

      c. Superficial surgery

B. Patient evaluation is aimed at identifying patients with coronary artery disease (CAD) or left ventricular dysfunction. Figure 30-1 is an algorithm for evaluating the patient's risk of developing a cardiac complication perioperatively. The history and physical examination can help identify factors that may increase a patient's risk of a cardiac complication during noncardiac surgery (Table 30-1). The **Goldman cardiac risk index** provides useful guidelines to help determine a patient's risk level (Table 30-2).

  1. Major predictors of increased perioperative risk

      a. Unstable coronary syndrome. Recent MI, active myocardial ischemia, and unstable angina each significantly increase the risk for an adverse cardiac outcome postoperatively.

      b. Decompensated CHF is a strong predictor of postoperative cardiac mortality and morbidity. The presence of a

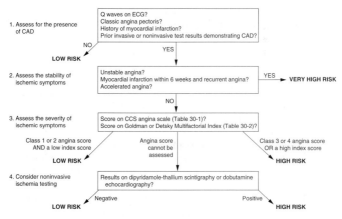

FIGURE 30-1. Algorithm for evaluating the patient's risk of developing coronary artery disease (CAD)-related complications following surgery. CCS = Canadian Cardiovascular Society; ECG = electrocardiogram; NYHA = New York Heart Association. (Modified with permission from Adler JS and Goldman L: Approach to the patient undergoing noncardiac surgery. In *Primary Cardiology*. Edited by Goldman L and Braunwald E. Philadelphia, WB Saunders, 1998, p 192.)

TABLE 30-1. Canadian Cardiovascular Society (CCS) Angina Scale

I Ordinary physical activity, such as walking and climbing stairs, does not cause angina. Angina occurs with strenuous or rapid or prolonged exertion at work or recreation.

II Slight limitation of ordinary activity. Angina occurs with walking or climbing stairs rapidly, walking uphill, walking or stair climbing after meals, or only during the few hours after awakening. Angina occurs when walking more than two blocks on the level or climbing more than one flight of stairs at a normal pace and in normal conditions.

III Marked limitation of ordinary physical activity. Angina occurs with walking one or two blocks on the level and climbing one flight of stairs in normal conditions and at a normal pace.

IV Inability to carry on any physical activity without discomfort; angina may be present at rest.

Reproduced with permission from Campeau L: Grading of angina pectoris. *Circulation* 54(3):522, 1976.

third heart sound (S_3), jugular venous distention, or peripheral edema should be assessed preoperatively. In general, all but emergent surgery should be postponed for patients with pulmonary edema.

    c. Severe arrhythmias [e.g., high-grade atrioventricular (AV) block, symptomatic ventricular tachycardia, or supraventricular tachycardia with rapid ventricular response] increase the cardiovascular risks of noncardiac surgery.

    d. Severe valvular disease, particularly severe aortic stenosis, identifies a patient as high risk. Mitral stenosis is associated with an increased risk for postoperative CHF. Aortic and mitral regurgitation are generally well tolerated postoperatively.

2. Intermediate predictors of increased perioperative risk

    a. Stable angina. Patients with mild stable angina whose functional capacity is normal should be able to tolerate surgery without further testing.

    b. Prior MI (identified by history or presence of pathologic Q waves) is accompanied by a reinfarction rate of about 6% for infarctions less than 3 months ago and a reinfarction rate of about 2% for infarctions 3–6 months ago. Elective surgery should generally be delayed in patients who have had an MI within the last 6 months.

    c. Compensated CHF is identified in patients with a reduced left ventricular ejection fraction, but no S_3, jugular venous distention, pulmonary edema, or peripheral edema.

TABLE 30-2. The Goldman Cardiac Risk Index

Step 1. Total the points for each criterion met by the patient:

Criteria	Points
Older than 70 years	5
MI within 6 months	10
S_3 gallop or elevated jugular venous distention	11
Severe aortic stenosis	3
A nonsinus ECG rhythm (other than PACs)	7
Greater than 5 PVCs per minute	7
Metabolic disease*	3
Intraperitoneal, intrathoracic, or aortic surgery	3
Emergency surgery	4

Step 2. Assess the patient's risk for a surgical complication:

Patient's Risk	Total Points	Risk of Death	Risk of a Life-Threatening Complication[†]
High	≥ 26	$\geq 20\%$	$\geq 20\%$
Intermediate	13–25	2%	10%–15%
Low-to-intermediate	6–12	$< 2\%$	5%
Low	≤ 5	$< 0.5\%$	$< 1\%$

ECG = electrocardiogram; MI = myocardial infarction; PAC = premature atrial contraction; PVC = premature ventricular complex; S_3 = third heart sound.

*Metabolic disease includes chronic liver disease, bedridden status, creatinine > 3.0 mg/dL, potassium < 3.0 meq/L or bicarbonate < 20 meg/L, $PO_2 < 60$ mm Hg, or $PCO_2 > 50$ mm Hg.

[†]Examples of life-threatening complications include myocardial infarction (MI), cardiogenic pulmonary edema, cardiac arrest and life-threatening arrhythmia.

These patients still have an increased risk of adverse cardiac events with surgery.

d. **Diabetes mellitus.** Patients with diabetes mellitus have an increased risk of silent ischemia, predisposing them to postoperative MI and CHF.

3. **Minor predictors of increased perioperative risk**
   a. **Older than 70 years**
   b. **Abnormal electrocardiographic findings,** such as left bundle branch block (LBBB), left ventricular hypertrophy (LVH), or nonspecific ST/T wave abnormalities
   c. **Nonsinus rhythm,** such as atrial fibrillation
   d. **Prior stroke**
   e. **Uncontrolled systemic hypertension**

C. **Preoperative cardiac diagnostic testing** is useful to help identify patients with high-risk CAD. If the history or physical examination reveals evidence of CAD, left ventricular dysfunction, or significant valvular disease, further cardiac testing should be considered before surgery.

HOT

KEY

Preoperative testing should only be used in patients in whom the results will change management.

---

1. **12-Lead electrocardiography** should be performed routinely in patients who are 40 years or older and in younger patients with risk factors, symptoms, or signs of cardiovascular disease. The electrocardiogram (ECG) may show evidence of prior MI, bundle branch block, LVH, arrhythmias, or ST/T wave changes associated with ischemia.
2. **Chest radiography** should be performed preoperatively in patients who are 40 years or older and in younger patients with risk factors, symptoms, or signs of cardiovascular disease. Cardiomegaly may signify left ventricular dysfunction. The chest radiograph may also provide a baseline if the patient develops postoperative CHF, pneumonia, or pulmonary embolism.
3. **Echocardiography** can be used to evaluate ventricular and valvular function in selected patients. It may also be appropriate for patients with suspected congenital heart disease.
4. **Noninvasive cardiac testing** can be used in patients with known or suspected coronary disease before high-risk surgery.
   a. The ability to exercise to the fourth stage of the Bruce treadmill test (i.e., longer than 9 minutes) is usually associated with a low perioperative cardiac event rate, even if electrocardiographic evidence of ischemia develops.
   b. Pharmacologic stress testing (e.g., dipyridamole, dobutamine) can be used in patients who cannot exercise.
5. **Coronary angiography** is useful in a small subset of patients before noncardiac surgery. Patients with severe or crescendo angina should be considered for coronary angiography and possible subsequent revascularization prior to elective high-risk surgery.

HOT

KEY

Coronary revascularization is appropriate prior to surgery if the patient has indications for revascularization, independent of the impending surgery.

III **PERIOPERATIVE MANAGEMENT.** Patients who are scheduled for noncardiac surgery frequently are being treated for cardiac disorders. Careful management of cardiac disease throughout the perioperative period is important to minimize the risks of a cardiac complication.

A. **CAD.** Antiplatelet and antianginal therapy generally should continue uninterrupted throughout the perioperative period. For patients who are not taking β blockers and do not have contraindications, **atenolol** (5–10 mg intravenously every 12 hours until able to take oral medications, followed by 50–100 mg orally once daily to complete a 7-day course) may reduce perioperative cardiac complications.

B. **CHF.** Careful attention to volume status is important. Consider intraoperative **hemodynamic monitoring** with a Swan-Ganz pulmonary artery (PA) catheter for patients with decompensated CHF.

C. **Hypertension.** Continuing antihypertensive medication is important.
   1. For patients with mild or moderate hypertension, nitropaste, nitropatch, or a clonidine patch may be used when the patient cannot take oral medications.
   2. For patients with severe hypertension, intravenous nitroglycerin (10–200 μg/min), hydralazine (10–40 mg every 6 hours), esmolol (50–300 μg/kg/min), or atenolol (5–10 mg every 12 hours) are useful perioperative agents.

D. **Tachyarrhythmias**
   1. **Atrial fibrillation or flutter.** Patients with a history of atrial fibrillation or flutter should be treated to adequately control the ventricular response perioperatively. Warfarin is usually discontinued 3 days before surgery, and restarted 1–2 days postoperatively.
   2. **Premature atrial contractions (PACs).** Frequent PACs (more than 5/hr) increase the risk for postoperative supraventricular tachycardias. Typically, no antiarrhythmic therapy is advocated. However, if the patient has a history of paroxysmal supraventricular tachycardia (PSVT), prophylactic β blocker or antiarrhythmic agents may be considered.
   3. **Premature ventricular complexes (PVCs).** Antiarrhythmic therapy generally should not be started during the perioperative period.
   4. **Ventricular tachycardia.** Patients with a history of ventricular tachycardia should be continued on antiarrhythmic therapy perioperatively. For those patients not receiving pharmacologic therapy, antiarrhythmics should not be started unless the patient meets the standard criteria for long-term treatment (see Chapter 9).

E. Bradyarrhythmias

1. **First degree AV block, Mobitz type I second degree block, and right bundle branch block (RBBB)** do not necessitate placement of a temporary transvenous pacemaker if the patient is asymptomatic. Agents that slow AV conduction (e.g., digoxin, β blockers, diltiazem, verapamil) should be avoided if possible.

2. **Mobitz type II second degree block, third degree AV block, and trifascicular block** (i.e., first degree AV block, RBBB, and left anterior or posterior fascicular block) signify high-risk AV block. Temporary pacing is indicated perioperatively, and permanent pacing may be indicated.

3. **LBBB.** A temporary pacemaker should be placed if a Swan-Ganz PA catheter is to be used.

F. Valvular disease. Antibiotic prophylaxis should be considered prior to high-risk surgery for patients with valvular disease.

1. **Severe aortic stenosis** increases the risk for perioperative pulmonary edema and arrhythmic death. Valve replacement or balloon valvuloplasty should be considered before elective surgery, particularly for symptomatic patients. Hemodynamic monitoring with a PA catheter is indicated.

2. **Aortic regurgitation** is generally well tolerated perioperatively. Hemodynamic monitoring may be considered for patients with severe aortic regurgitation.

3. **Severe mitral stenosis** increases the risk for perioperative pulmonary edema and life-threatening arrhythmias. Valve replacement or balloon valvuloplasty should be considered before surgery. Hemodynamic monitoring is important.

4. **Mitral regurgitation** is generally well-tolerated during surgery. A Swan-Ganz PA catheter may be used for patients with severe mitral regurgitation who are undergoing major surgery.

5. **Mechanical prosthetic valves.** Warfarin is generally discontinued 3 days before surgery. Unfractionated heparin may be started when the anticoagulation level becomes subtherapeutic.

IV POSTOPERATIVE TREATMENT OF CARDIAC COMPLICATIONS

A. Myocardial ischemia or infarction

1. **Presentation.** Because of the postoperative use of analgesics and sedatives, chest pain may not be present. Patients may instead present with heart failure, hypotension, arrhythmias, or altered mental status.

2. **Diagnosis.** Electrocardiographic changes and abnormal elevations in serum cardiac enzymes (e.g., troponin) lead to the diagnosis, which is supported by a new wall motion abnormality seen on echocardiography.

3. **Treatment.** Thrombolytics are generally contraindicated postoperatively; therefore, urgent coronary angiography and angioplasty are the treatment of choice. Additional therapy includes aspirin, β blockers, angiotensin-converting enzyme (ACE) inhibitors, and nitrates (see Chapter 13 V).

B. **CHF** may develop immediately or 3–5 days postoperatively as extracellular fluid is reabsorbed, thus increasing intravascular volume. Excluding MI by serial ECGs and cardiac enzyme measurements is important. Management primarily involves diuresis (e.g., furosemide). Afterload reduction (e.g., ACE inhibitors, hydralazine) and inotropic therapy (e.g., dopamine) may be added for selected patients.

C. **Blood pressure lability** is not uncommon postoperatively in patients with preexisting cardiovascular disease.

1. **Hypertension.** First determine whether pain control and fluid management are adequate. If significant hypertension is still present (i.e., systolic blood pressure > 200 mm Hg or diastolic blood pressure > 110 mm Hg), antihypertensive therapy may be administered as described in III C.

2. **Hypotension.** Consider serious causes of hypotension, including hypovolemia, cardiogenic shock, sepsis, adrenal insufficiency, and pulmonary embolism. Treatment may involve intravenous fluid boluses (e.g., normal saline 250–500 cc), followed by inotropic or vasopressor therapy (e.g., dopamine 5–20 μg/kg/min) if the hypotension persists.

D. **Arrhythmias.** Common causes of tachy- or bradyarrhythmias include electrolyte disturbances, hypoxemia, hyper- or hypovolemia, myocardial ischemia, heart failure, infection, and pulmonary embolism. Treatment (i.e., using antiarrhythmics or cardioversion for tachyarrhythmias and temporary transvenous pacing or atropine for bradyarrhythmias) is generally reserved for patients with significant arrhythmias accompanied by hypotension, heart failure, or myocardial ischemia.

E. **Pulmonary embolism** should be suspected in any patient who has unexplained dyspnea or chest pain postoperatively. If it is not contraindicated, intravenous heparin may be used. Consider placement of an umbrella filter in the inferior vena cava if anticoagulation therapy cannot be used. For patients with a massive pulmonary embolism, surgical embolectomy may be considered.

References

Detsky AS, Abrams HB, McLaughlin JR, et al: Predicting cardiac complications in patients undergoing non-cardiac surgery. *J Gen Intern Med* 1:211–219, 1986.

Eagle KA, Brundage BH, Chaitman BR, et al: Guidelines for perioperative cardiovascular evaluation for noncardiac surgery. Report of the American College of Cardiology/American Heart Association Task Force on Practice Guidelines (Committee on Perioperative Cardiovascular Evaluation for Noncardiac Surgery). *J Am Coll Cardiol* 27:910–948, 1996.

Fleisher LA, Eagle KA: Screening for cardiac disease in patients having noncardiac surgery. *Ann Intern Med* 124:767–772, 1996.

Mangano DT, Goldman L: Preoperative assessment of patients with known or suspected coronary disease. *N Engl J Med* 333:1750–1756, 1995.

Mangano DT, Layug EL, Wallace A, et al: Effect of atenolol on mortality and cardiovascular morbidity after noncardiac surgery. Multicenter Study of Perioperative Ischemia Research Group. *N Engl J Med* 335:1713–1720, 1996.

APPENDIX A. Equations and Parameters in Cardiology

Equations and Parameters	Normal Values
Hemodynamics:	
Central venous pressure (CVP)	0–8 mm Hg
Right ventricular systolic pressure	20–30 mm Hg
Right ventricular diastolic pressure	0–8 mm Hg
Pulmonary artery systolic pressure	20–30 mm Hg
Pulmonary artery diastolic pressure	10–15 mm Hg
Pulmonary artery mean pressure	15–20 mm Hg
Pulmonary capillary wedge pressure (PCWP)	8–12 mm Hg
Mean arterial pressure **(MAP)** = **[(SBP − DBP)/3] + DBP** where SBP = systolic blood pressure and DBP = diastolic blood pressure	80–100 mm Hg
Systemic vascular resistance **(SVR)** = **[(MAP − CVP) (80)]/CO** where CO = cardiac output	800–1200 dyne/sec/cm
Pulmonary vascular resistance **(PVR)** = **[(PAM − PCWP) (80)]/CO** where PAM = pulmonary artery mean pressure	40–120 dyne/sec/cm
PVR = [(PAM − PCWP)]/CO	0.5–1.5 Wood's units

Equations and Parameters	Normal Values

Cardiac Output and Oxygen-Carrying Capacity:

Cardiac output (**CO**) =
Heart rate × stroke volume

4–8 L/min

Fick CO (equation to estimate CO) =
[(3 ml/min) (kg)]/
[(SaO$_2$ − SvO$_2$) (13.9) (Hb)]
where SaO$_2$ = the oxygen saturation
in arterial blood

SvO$_2$ = the oxygen saturation in
venous blood
and Hb = hemoglobin (g/dL)

Cardiac index (**CI**) =
CO/BSA
where BSA = body surface area =
$\sqrt{[\text{height (cm)} \times \text{weight (kg)}/3600]}$

2.8–4.2 L/min/m^2

Arteriovenous oxygen difference
(**AV DO$_2$**) [to distinguish sepsis from
heart failure] = **arterial oxygen content (CaO$_2$)**
− venous oxygen content (CvO$_2$)

3.5–5

Arterial oxygen content (**CaO$_2$**) =
(1.34) (Hb) (SaO$_2$) + (0.003) (PaO$_2$)
where PaO$_2$ = partial pressure of
oxygen in arterial blood

20 ml O$_2$/dL

Venous oxygen content (**CvO$_2$**) =
(1.34) (Hb) (SvO$_2$) + (0.003) (PvO$_2$)
where PvO$_2$ = partial pressure of
oxygen in mixed venous blood

15 ml O$_2$/dL

if AV DO$_2$ < 3.5: decreased
peripheral oxygen
consumption
(sepsis)

if AV DO$_2$ > 5: circulatory
insufficiency
with increased
peripheral
oxygen
consumption
(e.g., congestive
heart failure)

Equations and Parameters	Normal Values

Valve Calculations:

Gorlin equation for aortic valve area =
[CO/(SEP) (HR)]/
$$\frac{[CO/(SEP)(HR)]}{[(44.3)(\sqrt{\text{mean LV-Ao pressure gradient}})]}$$
where SEP = systolic ejection period
(sec/beat)
HR = heart rate
and LV-Ao = left ventricular-aortic

$> 2 \text{ cm}^2$

Hakki equation for aortic valve area =
$$\frac{CO}{\sqrt{\text{mean LV-Ao pressure gradient}}}$$

$> 2 \text{ cm}^2$

Gorlin equation for mitral valve area =
[CO/(DFP) (HR)]/
$$\frac{[CO/(DFP)(HR)]}{[(37.7)(\sqrt{\text{mean PCWP-LV diastolic gradient}})]}$$
where DFP = diastolic filling period
(sec/beat)

$> 4 \text{ cm}^2$

Electrocardiographic:

QTc = QT interval/($\sqrt{\text{RR interval}}$)
where QTc = corrected QT interval (sec)

0.38–0.42 sec

APPENDIX B. Cardiovascular Pharmacology

Drug	Dose	Dosage Available	Comments
ANGIOTENSIN-CONVERTING ENZYME (ACE) INHIBITORS			
Benazepril (Lotensin)	Initial: 5–10 mg po qd Maintenance: 20–40 mg po qd Maximum: 40 mg po bid	5, 10, 20, 40 mg	**Administration:** Give 1–2 hr before or after antacids. **Drug Interactions:** increase in serum lithium; increase in serum potassium with potassium-sparing diuretics; NSAIDs may attenuate ACE inhibitor effect **Adverse Effects:** CNS—headache (5%), dizziness (3%), fatigue (3%); *Pulmonary*—cough (3%) *GI*—nausea (1%); *Renal*—increase in BUN and creatinine (increased risk with bilateral renal artery stenosis or severe CHF) **Warnings:** Contraindicated in patients who are pregnant, who have a history of angioneurotic edema, or who have severe bilateral renal artery stenosis. Monitor renal function and potassium levels closely.
Captopril (Capoten)	Initial: 6.25–25 mg po tid Maintenance: 50–100 mg po tid Maximum: 150 mg po tid	12.5, 25, 50, 100 mg	See benazepril

Drug	Dosing	Available forms	Pregnancy
Enalapril (Vasotec)	Initial: 2.5–5 mg po qd Maintenance: 10–20 mg po qd Maximum: 20 mg po bid	2.5, 5, 10, 20 mg	See benazepril
Enalaprilat (Vasotec IV)	Initial: 1.25 mg IV q6h Maximum: 5 mg IV q6h		See benazepril
Fosinopril (Monopril)	Initial: 5–10 mg po qd Maintenance: 20–40 mg po qd Maximum: 40 mg po bid	10, 20 mg	See benazepril
Lisinopril (Prinvil, Zestril)	Initial: 5–10 mg po qd Maintenance: 20–40 mg po qd Maximum: 40 mg po bid	2.5, 5, 10, 20, 40 mg	See benazepril
Moexipril (Univasc)	Initial: 7.5 mg po qd Maximum: 30 mg po qd	7.5, 15 mg	See benazepril
Perindopril (Aceon)	Initial: 2 mg po qd Maximum: 16 mg po qd	2, 4, 8 mg	See benazepril
Quinapril (Accupril)	Initial: 5–10 mg po qd Maintenance: 20–40 mg po dq Maximum: 40 mg po bid	5, 10, 20, 40 mg	See benazepril
Ramipril (Altace)	Initial: 2.5 mg po qd Maintenance: 5–10 mg po qd Maximum: 10 mg po bid	1.25, 2.5, 5, 10 mg	See benazepril

Drug	Dose	Dosage Available	Comments
Trandolapril (Mavik)	Initial: 1 mg po qd Maintenance: 2–4 mg po qd Maximum: 4 mg po bid	1, 2, 4 mg	See benazepril
ANGIOTENSIN II ANTAGONISTS			
Candesartan cilexetil (Atacand)	Initial: 16 mg po qd Maximum: 32 mg po qd	4, 8, 16, 32 mg	**Adverse Effects:** *CNS*—dizziness (3%); *GI*—diarrhea (2%); *Pulmonary*—cough (3%) **Warnings:** Contraindicated in patients who are pregnant or who have severe bilateral renal artery stenosis. Monitor renal function and potassium levels closely if the patient has a history of renal dysfunction.
Irbesartan (Avapro)	Initial: 75 mg po qd Maximum: 300 mg po qd	75, 150, 300 mg	See candesartan cilexetil
Losartan (Cozaar)	Initial: 25–50 mg po qd Maintenance: 50–100 mg po qd Maximum: 75 mg po bid	25, 50, 100 mg	See candesartan cilexetil
Telmisartan (Micardis)	Initial: 40 mg po qd Maximum: 80 mg po qd	40, 80 mg	See candesartan cilexetil
Valsartan (Diovan)	Initial: 40–80 mg po qd Maximum: 160 mg po bid	80, 160 mg	See candesartan cilexetil

ANTI-ADRENERGIC AGENTS

Peripheral Alpha-Adrenergic Blockers

Doxazosin
(Cardura)

Initial: 1 mg po qhs
Maintenance: 2–4 mg po qd
Maximum: 8 mg po bid

1, 2, 4, 8 mg

Adverse Effects: *CV*—postural hypotension (1%); *CNS*—dizziness (19%), headache (14%); *Other*—edema (4%), sexual dysfunction (2%)

Prazosin
(Minipress)

Initial: 1 mg po qhs
Maintenance: 2–5 mg bid
Maximum: 10 mg po bid

1, 2, 5 mg

See doxazosin

Terazosin
(Hytrin)

Initial: 1 mg po qhs
Maintenance: 1–5 mg po qd
Maximum: 10 mg po bid

1, 2, 5, 10 mg

See doxazosin

Central Alpha-Adrenergic Agonists

Clonidine

Oral
(Catapres)

Initial: 0.1 mg po bid
Maximum: 0.6 mg po tid

0.1, 0.2, 0.3 mg

Transdermal
(Catapres-TTS)

1 patch every week

0.1, 0.2, 0.3
mg/day

Administration: When oral therapy is to be discontinued reduce the dose gradually over 2–4 days to avoid rebound hypertension.

Drug Interactions: Doxazosin, TCAs, and MAO inhibitors may decrease antihypertensive effect; may cause CNS depression when combined with alcohol, phenothiazines, barbiturates, or benzodiazepines

Adverse Effects: *CV*—postural hypotension (5%); *CNS*—delirium, drowsiness, hallucinations, headache (5%); *Other*—dry mouth (10%), rash (2%), sexual dysfunction (3%)

Drug	Dose	Dosage Available	Comments
Guanabenz (Wytensin)	Initial: 2–4 mg po bid Maximum: 32 mg po bid	4, 8 mg	See clonidine
Methyldopa Oral (Aldomet) IV	Initial: 250 mg po bid Maintenance: 250–500 mg po tid Maximum: 1 g po tid 250–500 mg qd (up to 1 g IV q6h)	250 mg/5 ml suspension; 125, 250, 500 mg	**Drug Interactions:** increase in serum lithium; TCAs or phenothiazines may decrease antihypertensive effect; use with caution with MAO inhibitors; decrease in absorption with iron **Adverse Effects:** *CV*—postural hypotension, bradycardia, sodium retention (5%); *CNS*—drowsiness, psychosis, depression (10%); *GI*—nausea, diarrhea (5%); *Hematologic*—positive Coombs tests (10%–20%); *Hepatic*—abnormal liver function tests (5%); *Other*—sexual dysfunction (5%), gynecomastia (2%), drug-induced fever (2%), positive lupus and rheumatoid factor (2%)

Peripheral Alpha-Adrenergic Agonists

Drug	Dose	Dosage Available	Comments
Guanadrel (Hylorel)	Initial: 5 mg po bid Maintenance: 20–40 mg po bid	10, 25 mg	**Drug Interactions:** TCAs, phenothiazines, and MAO inhibitors may decrease antihypertensive effect **Adverse Effects:** *CNS*—depression, drowsiness, fatigue, headache (10%); *GI*—nausea, increased motility (5%); *Other*—edema (3%) **Warnings:** Contraindicated in patients with suspected pheochromocytoma and in those who are using MAO inhibitors.

Guanethidine
(Ismelin)

Initial: 10 mg po qd
Maintenance: 25–50 mg po qd

10, 25 mg

See guanadrel

Reserpine
(Serpasil, Serpalan)

Initial: 0.05–0.1 mg po qd
Maintenance: 0.1–0.25 mg po qd

0.1, 0.25, 1 mg

Drug Interactions/Adverse Effects:
See guanadrel
Warnings: Contraindicated in patients with mental depression, peptic ulcer disease, or ulcerative colitis.

ANTIARRHYTHMIC AGENTS

Adenosine
(Adenocard)

6 mg IVB (3 mg from central line); may repeat twice with 12-mg dose

Drug Interactions: Caffeine and theophylline may decrease adenosine effect; dipyridamole may increaseadenosine effect
Adverse Effects: Transient chest pressure, dyspnea, flushing (up to 50%)

Amiodarone
Oral
(Cordarone, Pacerone)
[Class III]

200 mg po qd (up to 400 mg po qid); may give a loading dose until 10 g total, then 200–400 mg po qd

200 mg

Drug Interactions: Associated with an increase in serum levels when combined with digoxin, flecainide, procainamide, quinidine, or theophylline; may increase prothrombin time with warfarin

Drug	Dose	Dosage Available	Comments
IV	150 mg IV over 10 min, then 1 mg/min IVD for 6 hr, then 0.5 mg/min IVD; may give repeat boluses of 150 mg IV over 10 min prn		**Adverse Effects:** Dose-related *CV*—CHF (3%), bradycardia; *CNS*—tremor (10%); *GI*—nausea (15%), abnormal liver function tests (5%); *Dermatology*—blue skin discoloration (1%); *Endocrine*—hyperthyroidism or hypothyroidism (5%); *Pulmonary*—inflammation or fibrosis (2%)
Atropine	Initial: 0.5–1 mg IVB or ET Maximum: 1 mg tid		**Adverse Effects:** *CV*—severe bradycardia (5%); *CNS*—headache (5%), dizziness (5%); *Other*—dry mouth (15%), tremor (3%), dry hot skin (3%)
Bretylium (Bretylol) [Class IV]	Initial: 5 mg/kg IVB; may repeat with 10 mg/kg IVB followed by 2 mg/min IVD		**Drug Interactions:** Avoid if digoxin toxicity is suspected. **Adverse Effects:** *CV*—hypotension **Warnings:** Reduce dose for patients with renal impairment.
Digoxin Oral (Lanoxin) Elixir	Initial: 0.125–0.25 mg po qd	0.125, 0.25, 0.5 mg 0.05 mg/ml	**Drug Interactions:** Quinidine, verapamil, propafenone, and amiodarone may increase digoxin levels; barbiturates, phenytoin, and rifampin may decrease digoxin metabolism; cholestyramine and antacids may decrease GI absorption

Drug	Dosage	Form	Notes
IV	0.25 mg IV q6h for 1 mg total loading dose.		**Adverse Effects:** Toxicity suspected by CNS—hallucinations, visual disturbances, lightheadedness; CV—AV dissociation, atrial tachycardia, ventricular tachycardia, accelerated junctional rhythm, AV block; GI—nausea, diarrhea **Warnings:** Avoid IV calcium in digitalized patients. Reduce the dose in patients with renal impairment.
Digoxin-Immune Fab (Digibind)	2–20 vials IV (for digoxin toxicity) Number of vials = serum digoxin $(ng/ml) \times kg \times 0.0093$.	40 mg/vial	**Adverse Effects:** severe hypokalemia (5%)
Disopyramide (Norpace) [Class IA]	100–150 mg po qid	100, 150 mg	**Drug Interactions:** Erythromycin and quinidine may increase the levels of disopyramide. Phenytoin and rifampin may decrease the levels of disopyramide.
Sustained-release (Norpace CR)	200–300 mg po bid	100, 150 mg	
Flecainide (Tambocor) [Class IC]	Initial: 50–100 mg po bid Maximum: 200 mg po bid	50, 100, 150 mg	**Drug Interactions:** Amiodarone and cimetidine may increase levels of flecainide. Flecainide may increase digoxin levels. **Warnings:** Avoid in patients with structural heart disease.

Drug	Dose	Dosage Available	Comments
Ibutilide (Covert) [Class III]	0.01 mg/kg up to 1 mg IV over 10 min; may repeat dose if no response after 10 more minutes		**Administration:** Used in patients with atrial fibrillation or flutter. **Adverse Effects:** QT prolongation, torsade de pointes (< 8%) **Warnings:** Avoid in patients with hypokalemia or a prolonged QT interval.
Lidocaine [Class IB]	50–100 mg IV over 1–2 min; may rebolus after 5 min, followed by 1–4 mg/min IVD		**Adverse Effects:** CNS—nervousness, confusion, mood changes, tremor (5%); CV—hypotension, bradycardia(3%)
Mexiletine (Mexitil) [Class IB]	Initial: 200 mg po tid Maximum: 250 mg po qid	150, 200, 250 mg	**Drug Interactions:** May decrease mexiletine levels when combined with antacids, narcotics, phenytoin, and rifampin; may increase theophylline levels **Adverse Effects:** CV—proarrhythmia (3%); CNS—lightheadedness, nervousness, headache (3%); GI—nausea, diarrhea (3%); Hematologic—agranulocytosis (0.06%), thrombocytopenia (0.16%)
Moricizine (Ethmozine) [Class IC]	Initial: 200 mg po tid Maximum: 300 mg po tid	200, 250, 300 mg	**Drug Interactions:** Cimetidine may increase levels of moricizine. Theophylline may decrease levels of moricizine. **Adverse Effects:** CV—proarrhythmia (3%)

Procainamide
Oral
(Procan SR,
Pronestyl-SR)
Extended-
release
(Procanbid)
[Class IA]
IV

500–1000 mg po qid

250, 500, 750,
1000 mg

500–1000 mg po bid

500, 1000 mg

17 mg/kg IVB over 1 hr,
then 2–4 mg/min IVD

Drug Interactions: Propranolol, cimetidine, ranitidine, quinidine, trimethoprim, and amiodarone may increase levels of procainamide.
Adverse Effects: CV—hypotension (5%), proarrhythmia (3%); CNS—depression, psychosis (2%); GI—nausea,diarrhea (3%); Hematologic—neutropenia (< 1%), thrombocytopenia (< 1%)

Propafenone
(Rythmol)
[Class IC]

Initial: 150 mg po tid
Maximum: 300 mg po tid

150, 225, 300 mg

Drug Interactions: Cimetidine and quinidine may increase levels of propafenone. Propafenone may increase levels of digoxin and cyclosporine.
Adverse Effects: See procainamide

Quinidine gluconate
(Quinaglute,
Quinalan)
[Class IA]

324 mg po every 8–12 hr

324 mg

Drug Interactions: Amiodarone, antacids, cimetidine, verapamil, TCAs, and β blockers may increase levels of quinidine. Barbiturates, nifedipine, sucralfate, phenytoin, and rifampin may decrease levels of quinidine. Quinidine may increase levels of digoxin, procainamide, propafenone, and disopyramide.
Adverse Effects: Diarrhea (10%), nausea (5%), depression (3%)

Drug	Dose	Dosage Available	Comments
Quinidine sulfate (Quinidex, Quinora)	300–600 mg po every 8–12 hr	300 mg	See quinidine gluconate
Sotalol (Betapace) [Class III]	Initial: 40–80 mg po bid Maximum: 640 mg/day	80, 120, 160, 240 mg	**Adverse Effects:** CV—proarrhythmia (3%), excessive bradycardia (3%)
Tocainide (Tonocard) [Class IB]	200–600 mg po tid	400, 600 mg	**Drug Interactions:** Rifampin and cimetidine may decrease levels of tocainide. Allopurinol may increase levels of tocainide.
ANTIPLATELET AGENTS			
Abciximab (ReoPro)	0.25 mg/kg IVB followed by 10 μg/min IVD for 12 hr		**Action:** Glycoprotein IIb/IIIa inhibitor **Adverse Effects:** hemorrhage, bleeding complications **Warnings:** Platelet transfusion may be indicated if severe hemorrhagic complications arise.
Aspirin	81–325 mg po qd	81, 325 mg	**Adverse Effects:** GI—dyspepsia, nausea, gastrointestinal bleeding (rare)
Clopidogrel (Plavix)	75 mg po qd	75 mg	**Adverse Effects:** Dyspepsia and nausea (rare); extremely rare incidence of significant hematologic effects

Dipyridamole
Oral (Persantine)
Extended-release

75–100 mg po qid

25, 50, 75 mg

Adverse Effects: Minimal lightheadedness, headache, diarrhea, rash

Aggrenox (i.e., dipyridamole and aspirin)

1 tablet po qd

200/25 mg

Eptifibatide
(Integrilin)

Dose for acute coronary syndrome: 180 μg/kg IVB followed by 2 μg/kg/min IVD up to 72 hours

Dose for angioplasty: 180 μg/kg IVB followed by 2 μg/kg/min IVD for 18 hr, and give a second 180 μg/kg IVB 10 min after first bolus

Administration: Give with IV heparin to patients undergoing high-risk angioplasty or who have non-Q-wave MI.

Action: Glycoprotein IIb/IIIa inhibitor

Adverse Effects: See abciximab; may perform hemodialysis to reduce drug levels if severe hemorrhagic complications arise

Warnings: Avoid in patients with a serum creatinine > 4 mg/dl. In patients with a creatinine 2–4 mg/dl, reduce IVD by 50%.

Ticlopidine
(Ticlid)

250 mg po bid

250 mg

Drug Interactions: Ticlopidine may decrease levels of digoxin and increase levels of cimetidine and theophylline. Antacids may decrease ticlopidine absorption

Adverse Effects: *GI*—diarrhea (12%), dyspepsia (7%); *Hematologic*—neutropenia (2%), thrombotic thrombocytopenic purpura (rare)

Drug	Dose	Dosage Available	Comments
Tirofiban (Aggrastat)	*Dose for acute coronary syndromes:* 0.4 µg/kg/min for 30 min, followed by 0.1 µg/kg/min IVD for next 48–96 hr *Dose for angioplasty:* 10 µg/kg IVB over 3 min, followed by 0.15 µg/kg/min IVD for next 18 hr		See eptifibatide
ANTICOAGULANTS			
Coumadin (Warfarin)	1–10 mg po qhs	1, 2, 2.5, 3, 4, 5, 6, 7.5, 10 mg	**Drug Interactions:** Increased prothrombin response when combined with alcohol, allopurinol, amiodarone, cimetidine, fluoroquinolones, NSAIDs, lovastatin, methyldopa, metronidazole, phenytoin, propafenone, quinidine, quinine, ranitidine, tamoxifen, tolbutamide, and sulfa agents. Decreased prothrombin response when combined with adrenocortical steroids, antacids, carbamazepine, cholestyramine, haloperidol, nafcillin, oral contraceptives, rifampin, and trazodone. **Adverse Effects:** Bleeding, hemorrhage, skin necrosis

Enoxaparin
(Lovenox)

For non-Q-wave MI:
1 mg/kg SQ bid
For DVT prophylaxis:
30 mg SQ bid

Adverse Effects: Hemorrhage, thrombocytopenia
(2%)
Warnings: Use with caution in patients with renal
impairment.

Dalteparin
(Fragmin)

For DVT prophylaxis:
2500–5000 units SQ qd

Adverse Effects: See enoxaparin

Heparin

*For venous or arterial
thromboembolism:* 80
units/kg IVB, then 15–20
units/kg/hr IVD
For DVT prophylaxis:
5000 units SQ every
8–12 hr

Adverse Effects: Hemorrhage, thrombocytopenia
(2%–5%), cutaneous necrosis

Lepirudin
(Refludan)

*For heparin-associated
thrombocytopenia:*
0.4 mg/kg IVB, then
0.15 mg/kg/hr IVD

Adverse Effects: See enoxaparin

ANTIHYPERTENSIVE AGENTS—OTHER

Epoprostenol
(Flolan)

2 ng/kg/min IVD, titrate up
to 16 ng/kg/min IVD for
patients with pulmonary
hypertension

Action: Prostacyclin agonist
Administration: Given via central line
Adverse Effects: Dose-related flushing, headache,
nausea, palpitations, lightheadedness

273

Drug	Dose	Dosage Available	Comments
Fenoldopam (Corlopam)	0.03–0.3 µg/kg/min IVD for as long as 48 hr		**Action:** Selective D₁-dopamine receptor agonist
Hydralazine (Apresoline)	Initial: 10 mg po qid; 10 mg IV or IM every 4–6 hr Maximum: 100 mg po tid	10, 25, 50, 100 mg	**Adverse Effects:** *CV*—palpitations, tachycardia; *CNS*—headache; *Rheumatologic*—SLE with high doses (> 200 mg/day)
Minoxidil (Loniten)	Initial: 5 mg po qd Maximum: 30 mg po tid	2.5, 10 mg	**Adverse Effects:** Hypertrichosis (80%); edema (7%)
Nitroprusside (Nipride)	Initial: 0.3 µg/kg/min IV Maximum: 10 µg/kg/min IVD, or 3.5 mg/kg total dose *For cyanide toxicity:* 3% sodium nitrate 5 mg/kg over 2–4 min IV, followed by sodium thiosulfate 150–250 mg/kg IV		**Adverse Effects:** Cyanide and thiocyanate toxicity (air hunger, confusion, lactic acidosis, bright red venous blood), methemoglobinemia. **Warnings:** Reduce the dose in the elderly or in patients with hepatic or renal impairment.
Phentolamine (Regitine)	*For pheochromocytoma:* 5 mg IV or IM in increments		**Administration:** Inject 5–10 mg of phentolamine in a 10 ml NaCl solution into affected area for cases of extravasation necrosis.

ANTIHYPERTENSIVE COMBINATIONS

Aldactazide (i.e., HCTZ and spironolactone) — 1–2 tablets po qd — 25 mg/25 mg, 50 mg/50 mg

Aldoclor (i.e., chlorothiazide and methyldopa) — 1 tablet po every 6–8 hr — 150/250 mg, 250/250 mg

Aldoril (i.e., HCTZ and methyldopa) — 1 tablet po tid — 15/250 mg, 25/250 mg, 30/500 mg, 50/500 mg

Apresazide (i.e., HCTZ and hydralazine) — 1 tablet po bid — 25/25 mg, 50/50 mg, 50/100 mg

Capozide (i.e., HCTZ and captopril) — 1 tablet po bid — 15/25 mg, 25/25 mg, 15/50 mg, 25/50 mg

Combipres (i.e., chlorthalidone and clonidine) — 1 tablet po bid — 15/0.1 mg, 15/0.2 mg, 15/0.3 mg

Corzide (i.e., bendroflumethiazide and nadolol) — 1–2 tablets po qd — 5/40 mg, 5/80 mg

Diovan (i.e., HCTZ and valsartan) — 1–2 tablets po qd — 12.5/80 mg, 12.5/160 mg

Dyazide (i.e., HCTZ and triamterene) — 1–2 tablets po qd — 25/37.5 mg

Esimil (i.e., HCTZ and guanethidine) — 1–2 tablets po qd — 25/10 mg

Hyzaar (i.e., hydrochlorothiazide and losartan) — 1–2 tablets po qd — 12.5/50 mg

Inderide (i.e., HCTZ and propranolol) — 1–2 tablets po bid — 25/40 mg, 25/80 mg

Inderide LA (i.e., HCTZ and propranolol) — 1–2 tablets po qd — 50/80 mg, 50/120 mg, 50/160 mg

Lexxel (i.e., enalapril and felodipine) — 1–2 tablets po qd — 5/5 mg

Lopressor HCT (i.e., HCTZ and metoprolol) — 1 tablet po bid — 25/50 mg, 25/100 mg, 50/100 mg

Lotensin HCT (i.e., HCTZ and benazepril) — 1–2 tablets po qd — 6.25/5 mg, 12.5/10 mg, 12.5/20 mg, 25/20 mg

Lotrel (i.e., amlodipine and benazepril) — 1–2 tablets po qd — 2.5/10 mg, 5/10 mg, 5/20 mg

Maxzide (i.e., HCTZ and triamterene) — 1–2 tablets po qd — 25/37.5 mg, 50/75 mg

Minizide (i.e., polythiazide and prazosin) — 1–2 tablets po bid — 0.5/1 mg, 0.5/2 mg, 0.5/5 mg

Moduretic (i.e., HCTZ and amiloride) — 1–2 tablets po qd — 50/5 mg

Normozide (i.e., HCTZ and labetalol) — 1–2 tablets po bid — 25/100 mg, 25/200 mg, 25/300 mg

Prinzide (i.e., HCTZ and lisinopril) — 1–2 tablets po qd — 12.5/10 mg, 12.5/20 mg, 25/20 mg

Ser-Ap-Es (i.e., HCTZ, reserpine and hydralazine) — 1–2 tablets po tid — 15/0.1/25 mg

Tarka (i.e., trandolapril and verapamil) — 1–2 tablets po qd — 2/180 mg, 1/240 mg, 2/240 mg, 4/240 mg

Drug	Dose	Dosage Available	Comments
Teczem (i.e., enalapril and diltiazem CD)		1–2 tablets po qd	5/180 mg
Tenoretic (i.e, chlorthalidone and atenolol)		1–2 tablets po qd	25/50 mg, 25/100 mg
Timolide (i.e., HCTZ and timolol)		1–2 tablets po qd	25/10 mg
Trandate HCT (i.e., HCTZ and labetalol)		1–2 tablets po bid	25/100 mg, 25/200 mg, 25/300 mg
Uniretic (i.e., HCTZ and moexipril)		1–2 tablets po qd	12.5/7.5 mg, 25/15 mg
Vaseretic (i.e., HCTZ and enalapril)		1–2 tablets po qd	12.5/5 mg, 25/10 mg
Zestoretic (i.e., HCTZ and lisinopril)		1–2 tablets po qd	12.5/10 mg, 12.5/20 mg, 25/20 mg
Ziac (i.e., HCTZ and bisoprolol)		1–2 tablets po qd	6.25/2.5 mg, 6.25/5 mg, 6.25/10 mg
BETA-ADRENERGIC ANTAGONISTS			
Acebutolol (Sectral)	Initial: 200 mg po bid Maximum: 600 mg po bid	200, 400 mg	**Action:** β1 selective with ISA **Adverse Effects:** CV—bradycardia, CHF; *Endocrine*—hyperglycemia, may blunt sympathetic reaction to hypoglycemia; *Other*—sexual dysfunction, depression **Warnings:** Avoid in patients with decompensated systolic dysfunction or high-grade AV block. Use with caution in patients with bronchospasm, renal, and hepatic impairment.
Atenolol (Tenormin)	Initial: 25 mg po qd Maximum: 100 mg po qd	25, 50, 100 mg	**Action:** β1 selective **Adverse Effects/Warnings:** See acebutolol
Betaxolol (Kerlone)	Initial: 10 mg po qd Maximum: 20 mg po qd	10, 20 mg	**Action:** β1 selective **Adverse Effects/Warnings:** See acebutolol

276

Bisoprolol
(Zebeta)

Initial: 5 mg po qd
Maximum: 20 mg po bid

5, 10 mg

Action: β1 selective
Adverse Effects/Warnings: See acebutolol

Carteolol
(Cartrol)

Initial: 2.5 mg po qd
Maximum: 10 mg po qd

2.5, 5 mg

Action: Nonselective with ISA
Adverse Effects/Warnings: See acebutolol

Carvedilol
(Coreg)

Initial: 6.25 mg po bid
Maximum: 50 mg po bid

3.125, 6.25, 12.5, 25 mg

Action: Nonselective, α1 blocker, antioxidant, antiarrhythmic
Adverse Effects/Warnings: See acebutolol

Esmolol
(Brevibloc)

50–300 μg/kg/min IVD; may bolus with 250 mg/kg IV over 1 hr

Action: β1 selective
Adverse Effects/Warnings: See acebutolol

Labetalol

Oral
(Trandate, Normodyne)

Initial: 100 mg po bid
Maximum: 600 mg po qid

100, 200, 300 mg

Action: Nonselective, α1 blocker.
Adverse Effects/Warnings: See acebutolol

IV

Initial: 20 mg IVB every 10 min
Maximum: 300 mg IV over 24 hr

Metoprolol

Oral
(Lopressor)

Initial: 25 mg po bid
Maximum: 200 mg po bid

50, 100 mg

Action: β1 selective
Adverse Effects/Warnings: See acebutolol

Extended-release
(Toprol XL)

Initial: 50 mg qd
Maximum: 200 mg po bid

50, 100, 200 mg

IV

Initial: 5 mg IV every 5 minutes up to 15 mg IV

Drug	Dose	Dosage Available	Comments
Nadolol (Corgard)	Initial: 20 mg po qd Maximum: 160 mg po bid	20, 40, 80, 120, 160 mg	**Action:** Nonselective **Adverse Effects/Warnings:** See acebutolol
Penbutolol (Levatol)	Initial: 20 mg po qd Maximum: 40 mg po bid	20 mg	**Action:** Nonselective with ISA **Adverse Effects/Warnings:** See acebutolol
Pindolol (Visken)	Initial: 5 mg po bid Maximum: 20 mg po tid	5, 10 mg	**Action:** Nonselective with ISA **Adverse Effects/Warnings:** See acebutolol
Propranolol Oral (Inderal)	Initial: 10 mg po tid Maximum: 200 mg po tid	10, 20, 40, 60, 80, 90 mg; 4 and 8 mg/ml solution	**Action:** Nonselective **Adverse Effects/Warnings:** See acebutolol
Sustained-release (Inderal LA)	Initial: 60 mg po qd Maximum: 160 mg po bid	60, 80, 120, 160 mg	
IV	Initial: 1–3 mg IVB every 3 min Maximum: 1 mg/min IVD		
Timolol (Blocadren)	Initial: 5 mg po bid Maximum: 30 mg po bid	5, 10, 20 mg	**Action:** Nonselective with ISA **Adverse Effects/Warnings:** See acebutolol

CALCIUM CHANNEL ANTAGONISTS

Dihydropyridines

Amlodipine
(Norvasc)

Initial: 2.5–5 mg po qd
Maximum: 10 mg po qd

2.5, 5, 10 mg

Adverse Effects: CNS—headache (7%), lightheadedness (3%); CV—peripheral edema (10%)

Felodipine
(Plendil)

Initial: 5 mg po qd
Maximum: 10 mg po bid

2.5, 5, 10 mg

See amlodipine

Isradipine
Oral
(DynaCirc)
Sustained-release
(DynaCirc CR)

Initial: 2.5 mg po bid
Maximum: 10 mg po qd
Initial: 5 mg po qd
Maximum: 20 mg po qd

2.5, 5 mg

5, 10 mg

See amlodipine

Nicardipine
Oral
(Cardene)
Sustained-release
(Cardene SR)
IV

Initial: 20 mg po tid
Maximum: 40 mg po tid
Initial: 30 mg po bid
Maximum: 60 mg po bid

Initial: 5 mg/hr IVD
Maximum: 15 mg/hr IVD

20, 30 mg

30, 45, 60 mg

See amlodipine

Drug	Dose	Dosage Available	Comments
Nifedipine Oral (Procardia, Adalat) Sustained- release (Procardia XL, Adalat CC)	Initial: 10 mg po tid Maximum: 40 mg po tid Initial: 30 mg po qd Maximum: 60 mg po bid	10, 20 mg 30, 60, 90 mg	**Drug Interactions:** Cimetidine may increase bioavailability of nifedipine. Nifedipine may increase digoxin levels and decrease quinidine levels. **Adverse Effects:** CNS—headache (10%–20%), lightheadedness (4%–25%); CV—CHF (2%–7%), peripheral edema (7%–30%) **Warnings:** Avoid in patients with a history of CHF or MI.
Nisoldipine (Sular)	Initial: 10 mg po qd Maximum: 30 mg po bid	10, 20, 30, 40 mg	See amlodipine
Non-Dihydropyridines			
Diltiazem Oral (Cardizem) Sustained- release (Cardizem SR) Once-daily sustained- release (Cardizem CD, Dilacor XR, Tiazac)	Initial: 30 mg po qid Maximum: 90 mg po qid Initial: 60 mg po bid Maximum: 180 mg po bid Initial: 120 mg po qd Maximum: 240 mg po bid	30, 60, 90, 120 mg 60, 90, 120 mg 120, 180, 240, 300 mg; 360 mg (for Tiazac only)	**Drug Interactions:** Cimetidine and ranitidine may increase bioavailability of diltiazem. Diltiazem may increase digoxin, cyclosporine, and carbamazepine levels. **Adverse Effects:** CNS—headache (2%–10%), lightheadedness (2%–7%); CV—peripheral edema (2%–9%) **Warnings:** Avoid in patients with decompensated systolic dysfunction or high-grade AV block. Avoid also in patients with wide complex tachyarrhythmias and in those with atrial flutter or fibrillation conducting via an accessory pathway.

IV

Initial: 0.25 mg/kg IVB up to 20 mg IV over 2 min; may rebolus 15 min later with 0.35 mg/kg IVB up to 25 mg IV over 2 min; infuse 5–15 mg/hr IVD

Verapamil

Oral
(Calan, Isoptin)

Initial: 40 mg po tid
Maximum: 120 mg po tid

40, 80, 120 mg

Sustained-release
(Calan SR, Covera-HS, Isoptin SR, Verelan)

Initial: 120 mg po qd
Maximum: 240 mg po bid

120, 180, 240; 360 mg (for Verelan only)

IV

Initial: 0.1 mg/kg up to maximum of 10 mg IV over 2 min; may rebolus 30 min later with up to 10 mg IV over 2 min

Drug Interactions: Verapamil may decrease lithium levels and may increase levels of digoxin, cyclosporine, carbamazepine, and theophylline.

Adverse Effects: CNS—headache (2%), lightheadedness (3%); CV—peripheral edema (2%); GI—constipation (7%)

Warnings: See diltiazem

Drug	Dose	Dosage Available	Comments
DIURETICS			
Carbonic Anhydrase Inhibitors			
Acetazolamide (Diamox)	Initial: 125 mg po qd Maximum: 500 mg po tid	125, 250, 500 mg	**Warnings:** Use with caution in patients with hyponatremia, hypokalemia, adrenocortical insufficiency, or liver or renal dysfunction.
Dichlorphenamide (Daranide)	Initial: 50 mg po bid Maximum: 100 mg po bid	50 mg	See acetazolamide
Methazolamide (Neptazane)	Initial: 50 mg po bid Maximum: 100 mg po tid	50 mg	See acetazolamide
Loop Diuretics			
Bumetanide Oral (Bumex) IV/IM	Initial: 0.5 mg po qd Maximum: 3 mg po tid Initial: 0.5 mg IV or IM every 6 hours Maximum: 2.5 mg IV/IM qid	0.5, 1, 2 mg	**Drug Interactions:** May increase serum levels of digoxin and lithium; may increase the effect of anticoagulants **Adverse Effects:** Encephalopathy with preexisting liver disease, dry mouth, thrombocytopenia, hypokalemia, hypomagnesemia **Warnings:** Use with caution in patients with hypersensitivity to sulfonamides. Cross-reactivity is rare in patients with furosemide allergy.
Ethacrynic acid Oral (Edecrin) IV/IM	Initial: 25 mg po qd Maximum: 100 mg po bid Initial: 0.5–1 mg/kg up to 50 mg IV qd	25, 50 mg	**Drug Interactions:** May increase serum lithium levels; may increase anticoagulant effect of warfarin and ototoxicity of aminoglycosides and cisplatin **Adverse Effects:** See bumetanide

Drug	Dosage	Available Forms	Notes
Furosemide Oral (Lasix) IV	Initial: 20 mg po every morning Maximum: 160 mg po qid Initial: 10 mg IV every 6 hours Maximum: 80 mg IV every 6 hours	20, 40, 80 mg, solution 10 and 40 mg/5 ml	See ethacrynic acid
Torsemide Oral (Demadex) IV	Initial: 5 mg po qd Maximum: 100 mg po bid Initial: 5 mg IV qd Maximum: 20 mg IV qd	5, 10, 20, 100 mg	See ethacrynic acid

Potassium-Sparing Diuretics

Drug	Dosage	Available Forms	Notes
Amiloride (Midamor)	Initial: 5 mg po qd Maximum: 10 mg po bid	5 mg	**Adverse Effects:** *CNS*—headache (5%); *GI*—nausea, abdominal pain; *Hematologic*—aplastic anemia **Warnings:** Amiloride may cause severe hyperkalemia when used with ACE inhibitors or in patients with renal insufficiency.
Spironolactone (Aldactone)	Initial: 25 mg po qd Maximum: 200 mg po bid	25, 50, 100 mg	See amiloride

Drug	Dose	Dosage Available	Comments
Triamterene (Dyrenium)	Initial: 50 mg po bid Maximum: 150 mg po bid	50, 100 mg	See amiloride
Thiazide			
Benzthiazide (Exna)	Initial: 50 mg po qd Maximum: 200 mg po qd	50 mg	**Drug Interactions:** May increase levels of digoxin and lithium; may decrease absorption with cholestyramine **Adverse Effects:** Hypotension, vertigo, headache, nausea, interstitial nephritis, pancytopenia, photosensitivity, hemolytic anemia, Stevens-Johnson syndrome, hyperuricemia
Chlorothiazide Oral (Diuril) IV	Initial: 250 mg po qd Maximum: 1 g po bid Initial: 0.5 g IV qd Maximum: 1 g IV bid	*Tablets:* 250, 500 mg, *Suspension:* 250 mg/5 ml	See benzthiazide
Chlorthalidone (Hygroton)	Initial: 25 mg po qd Maximum: 100 mg po qd	15, 25, 50, 100 mg	See benzthiazide
Diazoxide (Hyperstat)	1–3 mg/kg up to 150 mg IV every 5 min		See benzthiazide

Hydrochloro-thiazide (HCTZ, Esidrix, HydroDIURIL, Microzide, Oretic)	Initial: 12.5 mg po qd Maximum: 100 mg po qd	*Tablets:* 25, 50, 100 mg *Solution:* 50 mg/5 ml	See benzthiazide
Indapamide (Lozol)	Initial: 1.25 mg po qd Maximum: 5 mg po qd	1.25, 2.5 mg	See benzthiazide
Methyclothiazide (Aquatensen, Enduron)	Initial: 2.5 mg po qd Maximum: 10 mg po qd	2.5, 5 mg	See benzthiazide
Metolazone (Zaroxolyn)	Initial: 2.5 mg po qd Maximum: 10 mg po bid	2.5, 5, 10 mg	Unlike other thiazides, metolazone is useful with creatinine clearance < 30 ml/min. **Drug Interactions/Adverse Effects:** See benzthiazide

HYPOLIPIDEMICS

Bile Acid Sequestrants

| **Cholestyramine** (Questran, Questran Light, Cholybar) Powder | 4 g po 1–6 times/day | | **Administration:** Mix powder in 4–6 oz of water, juice, or soup. Give 4–6 hr prior to or 1 hr after taking other medication.
Drug Interactions: May bind many drugs and impair GI absorption
Adverse Effects: *GI*—constipation (20%), bloating, flatulence, nausea |

Drug	Dose	Dosage Available	Comments
Colestipol (Colestid)			**Administration:** Mix powder in 4–6 oz of water, juice, or soup.
Tablets	Initial: 1 g po bid	1 g	**Drug Interactions/Adverse Effects:**
	Maximum: 4 g po qid		See cholestyramine
Granules	Initial: 5 g po bid	5 g/packet	
	Maximum: 5 g po six times daily		
HMG-CoA Reductase Inhibitors			
Atorvastatin (Lipitor)	Initial: 10 mg po qhs	10, 20, 40 mg	**Drug Interactions:** May increase anticoagulant effect when given with warfarin; increased risk of myopathy or rhabdomyolysis when given with cyclosporine, erythromycin, gemfibrozil, and niacin; may increase serum levels when given with cimetidine or omeprazole; may decrease serum levels when given with rifampin
	Maximum: 80 mg po qhs		
			Adverse Effects: CNS—dizziness, headache; GI—dyspepsia (8%); Hepatic—abnormal liver function tests (1%); Musculoskeletal—myalgia (1%–3%), myopathy (< 0.5%), rhabdomyolysis (rare).
			Warnings: Avoid in patients who are pregnant or nursing.

Drug	Dosage	Available Strengths	Drug Interactions/Adverse Effects/Warnings
Cerivastatin (Baycol)	Initial: 0.2 mg po qhs Maximum: 0.4 mg po qhs	0.2, 0.3, 0.4 mg	See atorvastatin
Fluvastatin (Lescol)	Initial: 20 mg po qhs Maximum: 40 mg po qhs	20, 40 mg	See atorvastatin
Lovastatin (Mevacor)	Initial: 10 mg po qhs Maximum: 80 mg po qhs	10, 20, 40 mg	See atorvastatin
Pravastatin (Pravachol)	Initial: 10 mg po qhs Maximum: 40 mg po qhs	10, 20, 40 mg	See atorvastatin
Simvastatin (Zocor)	Initial: 5 mg po qhs Maximum: 80 mg po qhs	5, 10, 20, 40, 80 mg	See atorvastatin
Other:			
Fenofibrate (TriCor)	Initial: 67 mg po qd (with meals) Maximum: 201 mg po qd	67 mg	**Drug Interactions:** May increase the effects of warfarin; increased risk of rhabdomyolysis when given with HMG-CoA reductase inhibitors **Adverse Effects:** GI—dyspepsia (20%), abdominal discomfort, diarrhea, abnormal liver function tests, gallstone formation **Warnings:** Avoid in patients with hepatic or severe renal dysfunction. Discontinue if the patient is pregnant or nursing, or if he has gallbladder disease, myositis, or hepatic disease.
Gemfibrozil (Lopid)	600 mg po bid	600 mg	**Administration:** Give 30 minutes before meals. **Drug Interactions/Adverse Effects/Warnings:** See fenofibrate

Drug	Dose	Dosage Available	Comments
Niacin Oral (Vitamin B3)	Initial: 100 mg po tid; double the dose weekly to reach goal dose of 1–2 g tid Maximum: 3 g tid	25, 50, 100, 250, 500 mg	**Administration:** Give with meals. Cutaneous flushing can be attenuated with aspirin pretreatment 20 minutes before the niacin dose. **Adverse Effects:** *GI*—dyspepsia; *Hepatic*—abnormal liver function tests; *Other*—flushing, hyperuricemia **Warnings:** The risk of rhabdomyolysis may increase slightly when niacin is given with HMG-CoA reductase inhibitors. Avoid sustained-release niacin because of the increased hepatotoxicity risk.
Extended-release (Niaspan) (Slo-Niacin)	Initial: 500 mg po qhs Maximum: 1000 mg po bid Initial: 250 mg po qhs Maximum: 2 g po qid	500 mg 250, 500, 750 mg	
NITRATES			
Isosorbide dinitrate (Isordil, Sorbitrate) Sustained-release (Isordil Tembids, Dilatrate SR)	Initial: 10 mg po tid Maximum: 80 mg po tid Initial: 40 mg po bid Maximum: 80 mg po bid	5, 10, 20, 30, 40 mg 40 mg	**Adverse Effects:** *CNS*—headache; *CV*—hypotension, tachycardia; *Other*—flushing
Isosorbide mononitrate (Ismo, Monoket) Extended-release (Imdur)	Initial: 20 mg po bid 7 hours apart Maximum: 40 mg po bid Initial: 30 mg po qd Maximum: 240 mg po qd	20 mg 30, 60, 120 mg	See isosorbide dinitrate

Nitroglycerin

Ointment, 2%
(Nitrol, NitroBid)

Initial: 0.5 inches tid
Maximum: 4 inches every 4 hr

Spray (Nitrolingual)

1–2 oral sprays prn

Sublingual (Nitrostat)

1 tablet SL; may repeat every 5 min twice prn | 0.15, 0.3, 0.4, 0.6 mg

Transdermal

1 patch 12–16 hr/day | Doses in mg/hr:

Deponit | 0.2, 0.4
Minitran | 0.1, 0.2, 0.4, 0.6
Nitro-Dur, Transderm-Nitro | 0.1, 0.2, 0.4, 0.6, 0.8
Nitrodisc | 0.2, 0.3, 0.4

**IV (Tridil,
Nitro-Bid IV)**

Initial: 5 µg/min IVD
Maximum: 200 µg/min IVD

See isosorbide dinitrate

For IV nitroglycerin: Alcohol intoxication and tolerance with prolonged therapy

For ointment and transdermal form: Dermatologic reactions (e.g., allergy, pruritus, vesicles)

INOTROPES/PRESSORS

Amrinone
(Inocor)

Initial: 0.75 mg/kg IV over 2 min, then 5–10 µg/kg/min IVD; may rebolus 30 min later with 0.75 mg/kg IV over 2 min
Maximum: 10 mg/kg/day

Action: Inotrope, phosphodiesterase inhibitor
Adverse Effects: *CV*—tachyarrhythmia (3%), hypotension (1%); *Hematologic*—thrombocytopenia (2%); *Other*—abnormal liver function tests (2%)

Dobutamine
(Dobutrex)

Initial: 2–10 µg/kg/min IVD
Maximum: 40 µg/kg/min IVD

Action: β1, β2 agonist
Drug Interactions: TCAs potentiate pressor effects.

289

Drug	Dose	Dosage Available	Comments
Dopamine (Intropin, Dopastat)	Initial: 2–10 μg/kg/min IVD Maximum: 20 μg/kg/min IVD		**Adverse Effects:** CV—tachyarrhythmia, tachycardia, hypotension (β2 effects), or hypertension (β1 effects) **Action:** α1, β1, β2 agonist **Drug Interactions:** MAO inhibitors potentiate vasopressor effects. TCAs decrease vasopressor effects.
Ephedrine	Initial: 10–25 mg slow IV push; additional doses every 5–10 min Maximum: 150 mg/day		**Action:** α, β1, β2 agonist
Epinephrine (Adrenalin)	For ventricular fibrillation, pulseless ventricular tachycardia, and asystole: 1 mg IV push every 3–5 min. If inadequate, consider intermediate dose (2–5 mg) or high dose (0.1 mg/kg) IV push every 3–5 min For bradycardia or hypotension: 2–10 mcg/min IVD		**Action:** α, β1, β2 agonist

Metaraminol
(Aramine)

For anaphylaxis: 0.1–0.5 mg SC or IM, repeating as needed every 20 min; or 0.1–0.25 mg IV over 5 min, repeating as needed every 10 min

2–10 mg SC or IM; or 0.5–5 mg IVB followed by 5 μg/kg/min IVD

Action: α, β1 agonist
Warnings: Use with caution in patients with sulphite allergy. Tachyphylaxis occurs with prolonged treatment.

Milrinone
(Primacor)

Initial: 50 μg/kg IV over 10 min followed by 0.375 μg/kg/min IVD
Maximum: 0.75 μg/kg/min IVD

Action: Inotrope, phosphodiesterase inhibitor
Adverse Effects: CV—tachyarrhythmias, hypotension; *Hematologic*—thrombocytopenia (0.5%)

Norepinephrine
(Levophed)

Initial: 2–4 μg/min IVD
Maximum: 20 μg/min IVD

Action: α, β1 agonist

Phenylephrine
(Neo-Synephrine)

Initial: 40 μg/min IVD; may add 50–100 μg IVB as needed
Maximum: 200 μg/min IVD.

Action: α agonist
Warnings: Use with caution in patients with sulphite allergy.

Drug	Dose	Dosage Available	Comments
THROMBOLYTICS			
Alteplase (t-PA, Activase)	*Front-loaded dose:* 15-mg IVB, then 0.75 mg/kg IVD up to 50 mg over 30 min, then 0.5 mg/kg IVD up to 35 mg over the next 60 min		**Administration:** Given with IV heparin. **Contraindications:** Bleeding diathesis; major surgery or trauma < 10 days; GI bleeding < 3 months; stroke < 6 months; CNS tumor, hemorrhage, aneurysm, or arteriovenous malformation; prolonged CPR > 10 min; pregnancy; severe uncontrolled hypertension (> 200/110 mm Hg); venous/arterial puncture to noncompressible site (e.g., internal jugular or subclavian)
Anistreplase (APSAC, Eminase)	30 units IV over 2–5 min		See alteplase
Reteplase (Retavase)	10 units IV over 2 min, repeat same dose in 30 min		See alteplase

		Administration: Given with IV or SQ heparin.
Streptokinase (Streptase, Kabikinase)	1.5 million units IV over 1 hr	**Contraindications:** See alteplase; also, prior streptokinase < 1 year
Tenecteplase (TNKase)	0.55 mg/kg IVB up to 50 mg over 5 sec	See alteplase
Urokinase (Abbokinase)	2 million units IV over 1 hr	See alteplase

---

ACE = angiotensin-converting enzyme; AV = atrioventricular; bid = twice a day; BUN = blood urea nitrogen; CHF = congestive heart failure; CNS = central nervous system; CPR = cardiopulmonary resuscitation; CV = cardiovascular; DVT = deep vein thrombosis; ET = endotracheal; GI = gastrointestinal; HCTZ = hydrochlorothiazide; IV = intravenous; IVB = intravenous bolus; IVD = intravenous drip; IM = intramuscular; ISA = intrinsic sympathomimetic activity; MAO = monoamine oxidase; MI = myocardial infarction; NSAIDs = nonsteroidal anti-inflammatory drugs; po = by mouth; prn = as needed; qd = every day; qhs = at bedtime; qid = four times a day; q6h = every 6 hours; SC = subcutaneous; SL = sublingual; SLE = systemic lupus erythematosus; SQ = subcutaneous; TCAs = tricyclic antidepressants; tid = three times a day.

APPENDIX C. Advanced Cardiac Life Support (ACLS) Algorithms from the American Heart Association (AHA), Year 2000

The American Heart Association has used the following classification system in which indications for a particular therapy or intervention are designated as:

Class I: Conditions for which there is evidence for and/or general agreement that a given treatment is beneficial, useful, and effective.

Class II: Conditions for which there is conflicting evidence and/or a divergence of opinion about the usefulness/efficacy of a treatment.

Class IIa. Weight of evidence/opinion is in favor of usefulness/efficacy.

Class IIb. Usefulness/efficacy is less well-established by evidence/opinion.

Class III. Conditions for which there is evidence and/or general agreement that a treatment is not useful/effective and in some cases may be harmful.

Class Indeterminate: Conditions for which there is insufficient evidence to assign a class designation to a particular treatment.

Reproduced with permission
Guidelines 2000 for Cardiopulmonary Resuscitation and Emergency Cardiovascular Care. *Circulation*, 102(8), 2000. Copyright American Heart Association

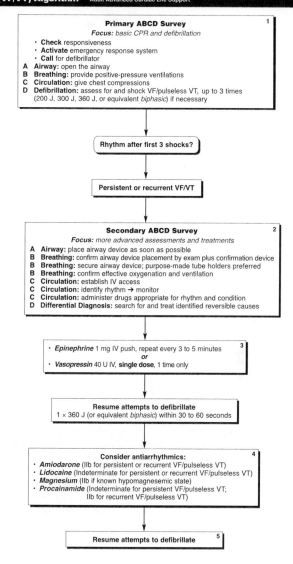

Primary ABCD Survey   1

Focus: basic CPR and defibrillation

- **Check** responsiveness
- **Activate** emergency response system
- **Call** for defibrillator

A **Airway:** open the airway
B **Breathing:** provide positive-pressure ventilations
C **Circulation:** give chest compressions
D **Defibrillation:** assess for and shock VF/pulseless VT, up to 3 times (200 J, 300 J, 360 J, or equivalent *biphasic*) if necessary

↓

Rhythm after first 3 shocks?

↓

Persistent or recurrent VF/VT

↓

Secondary ABCD Survey   2

Focus: more advanced assessments and treatments

A **Airway:** place airway device as soon as possible
B **Breathing:** confirm airway device placement by exam plus confirmation device
B **Breathing:** secure airway device; purpose-made tube holders preferred
B **Breathing:** confirm effective oxygenation and ventilation
C **Circulation:** establish IV access
C **Circulation:** identify rhythm → monitor
C **Circulation:** administer drugs appropriate for rhythm and condition
D **Differential Diagnosis:** search for and treat identified reversible causes

↓

- *Epinephrine* 1 mg IV push, repeat every 3 to 5 minutes   3
or
- *Vasopressin* 40 U IV, **single dose,** 1 time only

↓

Resume attempts to defibrillate
1 × 360 J (or equivalent *biphasic*) within 30 to 60 seconds

↓

Consider antiarrhythmics: 4
- *Amiodarone* (IIb for persistent or recurrent VF/pulseless VT)
- *Lidocaine* (Indeterminate for persistent or recurrent VF/pulseless VT)
- *Magnesium* (IIb if known hypomagnesemic state)
- *Procainamide* (Indeterminate for persistent VF/pulseless VT;
          IIb for recurrent VF/pulseless VT)

↓

Resume attempts to defibrillate   5

Notes for Ventricular Fibrillation (VF)/Pulseless Ventricular Tachycardia (VT) Algorithm

Assume that VF/VT persists after each intervention.

1

Defibrillatory shock waveforms

- Use **monophasic shocks** at listed energy levels (200 J, 300 J, 360 J) or **biphasic shocks** at energy levels documented to be clinically equivalent (or superior) to the monophasic shocks.

2

2A Confirm tube placement with

- Primary physical examination criteria *plus*
- Secondary confirmation device (end-tidal CO_2) [Class IIa]

2B Secure tracheal tube

- To prevent dislodgment, especially in patients at risk for movement, use purpose-made (commercially available) tracheal tube holders, which are superior to tie-and-tape methods (Class IIb)
- Consider cervical collar and backboard for transport (Class Indeterminate)
- Consider continuous, quantitative end-tidal CO_2 monitor (Class IIa)

2C Confirm oxygenation and ventilation with

- End-tidal CO_2 monitor *and*
- Oxygen saturation monitor

3

3A *Epinephrine* (Class Indeterminate) 1 mg intravenous (IV) push every 3 to 5 minutes. If this fails, higher doses of epinephrine (as much as 0.2 mg/kg) are acceptable but not recommended (there is growing evidence that it may be harmful).

3B *Vasopressin* is recommended only for VF/VT; there is no evidence to support its use in asystole or pulseless electrical activity (PEA). There is no evidence about the value of repeat vasopressin doses. There is no evidence about the best approach if there is no response after a single bolus of vasopressin. The following Class Indeterminate action is acceptable, but only on the basis of rational conjecture. If there is no response 5 to 10 minutes after a single IV dose of vasopressin, it is acceptable to resume epinephrine 1 mg IV push every 3 to 5 minutes.

Reproduced with permission
Guidelines 2000 for Cardiopulmonary Resuscitation and Emergency Cardiovascular Care. *Circulation*, 102(8), 2000. Copyright American Heart Association

4

4A *Antiarrhythmics* are indeterminate or Class IIb: acceptable; only fair evidence supports possible benefit of antiarrhythmics for shock-refractory VF/VT.

- *Amiodarone* (Class IIb) 300 mg IV push (cardiac arrest dose). If VF/pulseless VT recurs, consider administration of a second dose of 150 mg IV. Maximum cumulative dose: 2.2 g over 24 hours.
- *Lidocaine* (Class Indeterminate) 1.0 to 1.5 mg/kg IV push. Consider repeat in 3 to 5 minutes to a maximum cumulative dose of 3 mg/kg. A single dose of 1.5 mg/kg in cardiac arrest is acceptable.
- *Magnesium sulfate* 1 to 2 g IV in polymorphic VT (torsades de pointes) and suspected hypomagnesemic state.
- *Procainamide* 30 mg/min in refractory VF (maximum total dose: 17 mg/kg) is acceptable but not recommended because prolonged administration time is unsuitable for cardiac arrest.

4B *Sodium bicarbonate* 1 mEq/kg IV is indicated for several conditions known to provoke sudden cardiac arrest. See Notes in the Asystole and PEA Algorithms for details.

5

Resume defibrillation attempts: use 360-J (or equivalent biphasic) shocks after each medication or after each minute of cardiopulmonary resuscitation (CPR). Acceptable patterns: CPR-drug-shock (repeat) or CPR-drug-shock-shock-shock (repeat).

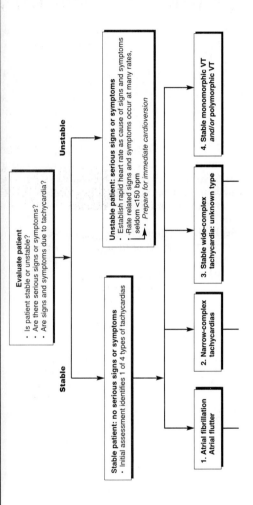

Tachycardia Algorithm
Adult Advanced Cardiac Life Support

Adult

Evaluate patient
- Is patient stable or unstable?
- Are there serious signs or symptoms?
- Are signs and symptoms due to tachycardia?

Stable

Unstable

Stable patient: no serious signs or symptoms
- Initial assessment identifies 1 of 4 types of tachycardias

Unstable patient: serious signs or symptoms
- Establish rapid heart rate as cause of signs and symptoms
- Rate related signs and symptoms occur at many rates, seldom <150 bpm
  - *Prepare for immediate cardioversion*

1. Atrial fibrillation
Atrial flutter

2. Narrow-complex tachycardias

3. Stable wide-complex tachycardia: unknown type

4. Stable monomorphic VT *and/or polymorphic VT*

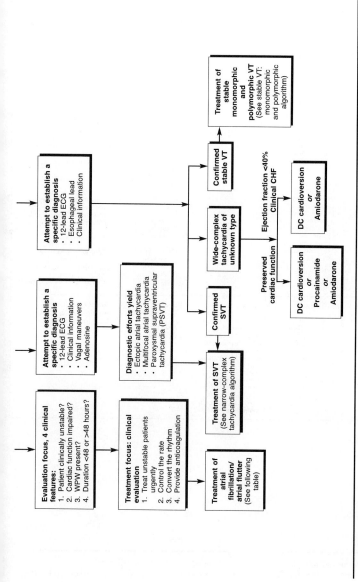

Evaluation focus, 4 clinical features:
1. Patient clinically unstable?
2. Cardiac function impaired?
3. WPW present?
4. Duration <48 or >48 hours?

Attempt to establish a specific diagnosis
• 12-lead ECG
• Clinical information
• Vagal maneuvers
• Adenosine

Attempt to establish a specific diagnosis
• 12-lead ECG
• Esophageal lead
• Clinical information

Treatment focus: clinical evaluation
1. Treat unstable patients urgently
2. Control the rate
3. Convert the rhythm
4. Provide anticoagulation

Diagnostic efforts yield
• Ectopic atrial tachycardia
• Multifocal atrial tachycardia
• Paroxysmal supraventricular tachycardia (PSVT)

Treatment of atrial fibrillation/atrial flutter
(See following table)

Treatment of SVT
(See narrow-complex tachycardia algorithm)

Confirmed SVT

Wide-complex tachycardia of unknown type

Confirmed stable VT

Treatment of stable monomorphic and polymorphic VT
(See stable VT: monomorphic and polymorphic algorithm)

Preserved cardiac function

Ejection fraction <40%
Clinical CHF

DC cardioversion
or
Procainamide
or
Amiodarone

DC cardioversion
or
Amiodarone

Control of Rate and Rhythm (Continued From Tachycardia Overview)

Atrial fibrillation/ atrial flutter with • Normal heart • Impaired heart • WPW	1. Control Rate		2. Convert Rhythm	
	Heart function preserved	**Impaired heart EF 40% or CHF**	**Duration <48 hours**	**Duration >48 hours or unknown**
Normal cardiac function	**Note:** *If AF >48 hours duration, use agents to convert rhythm with extreme caution in patients not receiving adequate anticoagulation because of possible embolic complications.* *Use only 1 of the following agents (see note below):* • Calcium channel blockers (Class I) • β-Blockers (Class I) • For additional drugs that are Class IIb recommendations, see Guidelines or ACLS text	*(Does not apply)*	**Consider** • DC cardioversion Use only 1 of the following agents (see note below): • Amiodarone (Class IIa) • Ibutilide (Class IIa) • Flecainide (Class IIa) • Propafenone (Class IIa) • Procainamide (Class IIa) • For additional drugs that are Class IIb recommendations, see Guidelines or ACLS text	• NO DC cardioversion! • **Note:** *Conversion of AF to NSR with drugs or shock may cause embolization of atrial thrombi unless patient has adequate anticoagulation.* • Use antiarrhythmic agents with extreme caution if AF >48 hours' duration *(see note above).* *or* ***Delayed cardioversion*** **Anticoagulation × 3 weeks at proper levels** • Cardioversion, *then* • Anticoagulation × 4 weeks more *or* ***Early cardioversion*** • Begin IV heparin at once • TEE to exclude atrial clot *then* • Cardioversion within 24 hours *then* • Anticoagulation ×4 more weeks
Impaired heart (EF <40% or CHF)	*(Does not apply)*	**Note:** *If AF >48 hours duration, use agents to convert rhythm with extreme caution in patients not receiving adequate anticoagulation because of possible embolic complications.* *Use only 1 of the following agents (see note below):* • Digoxin (Class IIb) • Diltiazem (Class IIb) • Amiodarone (Class IIb)	**Consider** • DC cardioversion *or* • Amiodarone (Class IIb)	• **Anticoagulation** as described above, followed by • **DC cardioversion**

Control of Rate and Rhythm (Continued From Tachycardia Overview)

Atrial fibrillation/ atrial flutter with • Normal heart • Impaired heart • WPW	1. Control Rate		2. Convert Rhythm	
	Heart function preserved	**Impaired heart EF 40% or CHF**	**Duration <48 hours**	**Duration >48 hours or unknown**

WPW	**Note:** *If AF >48 hours duration, use agents to convert rhythm with extreme caution in patients not receiving adequate anticoagula-tion because of possible embolic complications.*
	
	• DC cardioversion
	
	or
	
	• **Primary anti-arrhythmic agents** *Use only 1 of the following agents (see note below):*
	  • Amiodarone (Class IIb)
	  • Flecainide (Class IIb)
	  • Procainamide (Class IIb)
	  • Propafenone (Class IIb)
	  • Sotalol (Class IIb)
	
	-------------------- 	
	Class III (can be harmful)
	• Adenosine
	• β-Blockers
	• Calcium blockers
		• Digoxin
		Note: *If AF >48 hours duration, use agents to convert rhythm with extreme caution in patients not receiving adequate anticoagulation because of possible embolic complications.*
		
		• DC cardioversion
		
		or
		
		• Amiodarone (Class IIb)
			• DC cardioversion
			
			or
			
			• **Primary anti-arrhythmic agents** *Use only 1 of the following agents (see note below**):*
			  • Amiodarone (Class IIb)
			  • Flecainide (Class IIb)
			  • Procainamide (Class IIb)
			  • Propafenone (Class IIb)
			  • Sotalol (Class IIb)
			
			-------------------- 	
			Class III (can be harmful)
			• Adenosine
			• β-Blockers
			• Calcium blockers
			• Digoxin
				• **Anticoagulation** as described above, followed by
				• **DC cardioversion**

WPW indicates Wolff-Parkinson-White syndrome; AF, atrial fibrillation; NSR, normal sinus rhythm; TEE, transesophageal echocardiogram; and EF, ejection fraction.

Reproduced with permission
Guidelines 2000 for Cardiopulmonary Resuscitation and Emergency Cardiovascular Care. *Circulation,* 102(8), 2000. Copyright American Heart Association

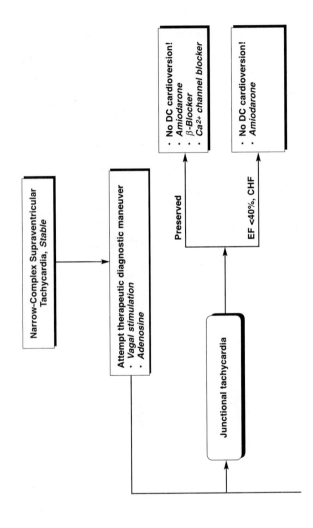

Narrow-Complex Supraventricular Tachycardia, *Stable*

Attempt therapeutic diagnostic maneuver
· *Vagal stimulation*
· *Adenosine*

Junctional tachycardia

Preserved

· **No DC cardioversion!**
· *Amiodarone*
· *β-Blocker*
· *Ca²⁺ channel blocker*

EF <40%, CHF

· **No DC cardioversion!**
· *Amiodarone*

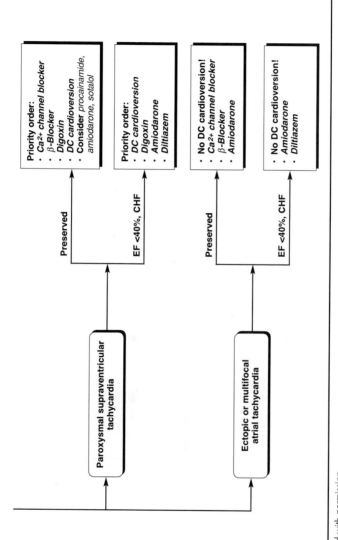

Paroxysmal supraventricular tachycardia

Preserved
Priority order:
· *Ca²⁺ channel blocker*
· *β-Blocker*
· *Digoxin*
· *DC cardioversion*
· *Consider* procainamide, amiodarone, sotalol

EF <40%, CHF
Priority order:
· *DC cardioversion*
· *Digoxin*
· *Amiodarone*
· *Diltiazem*

Ectopic or multifocal atrial tachycardia

Preserved
· No DC cardioversion!
· *Ca²⁺ channel blocker*
· *β-Blocker*
· *Amiodarone*

EF <40%, CHF
· No DC cardioversion!
· *Amiodarone*
· *Diltiazem*

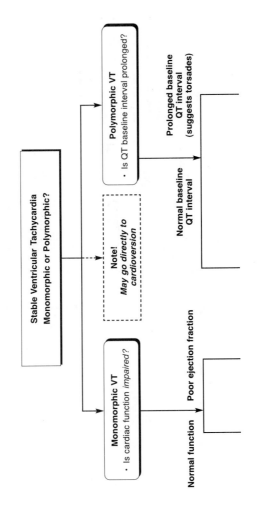

Stable Ventricular Tachycardia
Monomorphic or Polymorphic?

Note!
May go directly to cardioversion

Monomorphic VT
• Is cardiac function *impaired?*

Polymorphic VT
• Is QT baseline interval prolonged?

Normal function

Poor ejection fraction

Normal baseline QT interval

Prolonged baseline QT interval (suggests torsades)

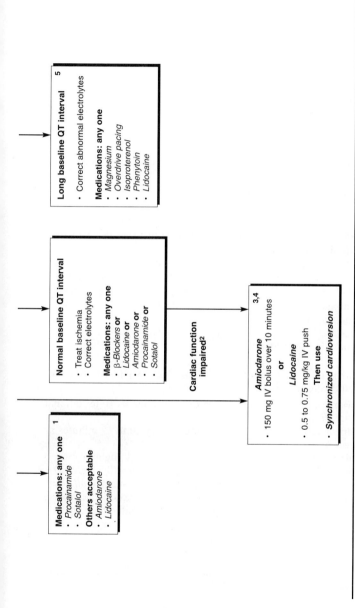

Medications: any one [1]
- Procainamide
- Sotalol

Others acceptable
- Amiodarone
- Lidocaine

Normal baseline QT interval
- Treat ischemia
- Correct electrolytes

Medications: any one
- β-Blockers **or**
- Lidocaine **or**
- Amiodarone **or**
- Procainamide **or**
- Sotalol

Cardiac function impaired[2]

Long baseline QT interval [5]
- Correct abnormal electrolytes

Medications: any one
- Magnesium
- Overdrive pacing
- Isoproterenol
- Phenytoin
- Lidocaine

Amiodarone [3,4]
- 150 mg IV bolus over 10 minutes

or

Lidocaine
- 0.5 to 0.75 mg/kg IV push

Then use
- *Synchronized cardioversion*

Notes for Stable Ventricular Tachycardia: Monomorphic or Polymorphic?

1

Monomorphic ventricular tachycardia (VT) with normal cardiac function

Use just 1 agent (to avoid proarrhythmic effects of combination therapy).

This reduces adverse side effects. Choose 1 agent from these lists:

Top agents

- Procainamide (IIa)
- Sotalol (IIa)

Other acceptable

- Amiodarone (IIb)
- Lidocaine (IIb)

2

Monomorphic or polymorphic ventricular tachycardia (VT) with impaired cardiac function

If clinical signs are suggestive of impaired left ventricle (LV) function (ejection fraction < 40% or congestive heart failure) in either long- or normal-QRS tachycardias, use

- Amiodarone (IIb)
- Lidocaine (IIb)

then use

- Synchronized cardioversion

3

Detailed dosing of amiodarone (Class IIb) in patients with impaired cardiac function

- 150 mg intravenous (IV) bolus over 10 minutes (international dose: 5 mg/kg)
- Repeat 150 mg IV (over 10 minutes) every 10 to 15 minutes as needed
- Alternative infusion: 360 mg over 6 hours (1 mg/min over 6 hours), then 540 mg over the remaining 18 hours (0.5 mg/min)
- Maximum total dose: 2.2 g in 24 hours. This means that *all* doses (including those used in resuscitation) should be added together, so the total cumulative dose per 24 hours is limited to 2.2 g

4

Detailed dosing of lidocaine (Class Indeterminate) in patients with impaired cardiac function

- 0.5 to 0.75 mg/kg IV push
- Repeat every 5 to 10 minutes
- Then infuse 1 to 4 mg/min
- Maximum total dose: 3 mg/kg (over 1 hour)

5

If rhythm is suggestive of torsades de pointes

- Stop/avoid treatments that prolong QT
- Identify and treat abnormal electrolytes

Medications (all Class Indeterminate):

- Magnesium
- Overdrive pacing (with or without β-blocker)
- Isoproterenol (as temporizing measure to overdrive pacing)
- Phenytoin or lidocaine

Reproduced with permission
Guidelines 2000 for Cardiopulmonary Resuscitation and Emergency Cardiovascular Care. *Circulation*, 102(8), 2000. Copyright American Heart Association

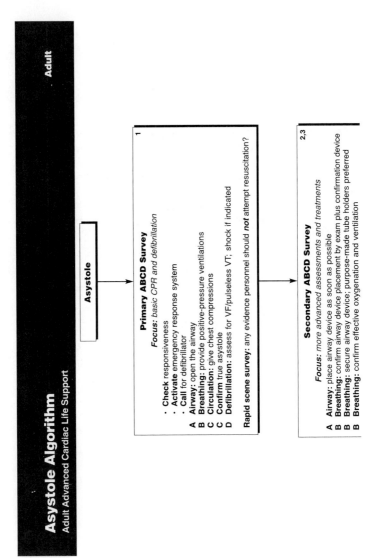

Asystole Algorithm
Adult Advanced Cardiac Life Support

Adult

Asystole

Primary ABCD Survey
Focus: basic CPR and defibrillation

- **Check** responsiveness
- **Activate** emergency response system
- **Call** for defibrillator
- **A Airway:** open the airway
- **B Breathing:** provide positive-pressure ventilations
- **C Circulation:** give chest compressions
- **C Confirm** true asystole
- **D Defibrillation:** assess for VF/pulseless VT; shock if indicated

Rapid scene survey: any evidence personnel should *not* attempt resuscitation?

1

Secondary ABCD Survey
Focus: more advanced assessments and treatments

- **A Airway:** place airway device as soon as possible
- **B Breathing:** confirm airway device placement by exam plus confirmation device
- **B Breathing:** secure airway device; purpose-made tube holders preferred
- **B Breathing:** confirm effective oxygenation and ventilation

2,3

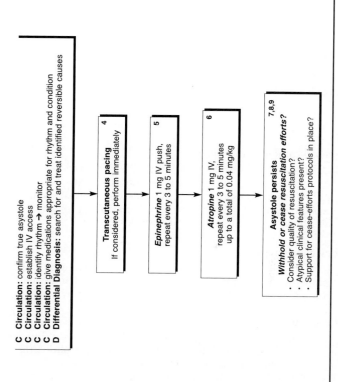

C **Circulation:** confirm true asystole
C **Circulation:** establish IV access
C **Circulation:** identify rhythm → monitor
C **Circulation:** give medications appropriate for rhythm and condition
D **Differential Diagnosis:** search for and treat identified reversible causes

4

Transcutaneous pacing
If considered, perform immediately

5

Epinephrine 1 mg IV push,
repeat every 3 to 5 minutes

6

Atropine 1 mg IV,
repeat every 3 to 5 minutes
up to a total of 0.04 mg/kg

7,8,9

Asystole persists
Withhold or cease resuscitation efforts?
• Consider quality of resuscitation?
• Atypical clinical features present?
• Support for cease-efforts protocols in place?

Reproduced with permission
Guidelines 2000 for Cardiopulmonary Resuscitation and Emergency Cardiovascular Care. *Circulation*, 102(8), 2000. Copyright American Heart Association

Notes for Asystole Algorithm

1

Scene Survey: DNAR (Do Not Attempt Resuscitation) patient?

If Yes: do not start/attempt resuscitation. Any *objective* indicators of DNAR status? Bracelet? Anklet? Written documentation? Family statements? If Yes: do not start/attempt resuscitation.

- Any *clinical* indicators that resuscitation attempts are not indicated (e.g., signs of death?) If Yes: do not start/attempt resuscitation.

2

Confirm true asystole

- Check lead and cable connections
- Monitor power on?
- Monitor gain up?
- Verify asystole in another lead?

3

Sodium bicarbonate 1 mEq/kg

- Indications for use include the following: overdose of tricyclic antidepressants; to alkalinize urine in overdoses; patients with tracheal intubation plus long arrest intervals; on return of spontaneous circulation if there is a long arrest interval.
- Ineffective or harmful in hypercarbic acidosis.

4

Transcutaneous pacing

- To be effective, must be performed early, combined with drug therapy. Evidence does not support routine use of transcutaneous pacing for asystole.

5

Epinephrine

- Recommended dose is 1 mg intravenous (IV) push every 3 to 5 minutes. If this approach fails, higher doses of epinephrine (as much as 0.2 mg/kg) may be used but are not recommended.
- We currently lack evidence to support routine use of vasopressin in treatment of asystole.

6

Atropine

- Use the shorter dosing interval (every 3 to 5 minutes) in asystolic arrest.

Reproduced with permission
Guidelines 2000 for Cardiopulmonary Resuscitation and Emergency Cardiovascular Care. *Circulation*, 102(8), 2000. Copyright American Heart Association

7

Review the quality of the resuscitation attempt

- Was there an adequate trial of BLS? of ACLS? Has the team done the following:
- Achieved tracheal intubation?
- Performed effective ventilation?
- Shocked ventricular fibrillation (VF) if present?
- Obtained IV access?
- Given epinephrine IV? atropine IV?
- Ruled out or corrected reversible causes?
- Continuously documented asystole > 5 to 10 minutes after all of the above have been accomplished?

8

Reviewed for atypical clinical features?

- Not a victim of drowning or hypothermia?
- No reversible therapeutic or illicit drug overdose
  —"Yes" to the questions in Notes 7 and 8 means the resuscitation team complies with recommended criteria to terminate resuscitative efforts where the patient lies (Class IIa)
  —If the response team and patient meet the above criteria, then withhold urgent field-to-hospital transport with continuing cardiopulmonary resuscitation (CPR) = Class III (harmful; no benefit)

9

Withholding or stopping resuscitative efforts out-of-hospital

If criteria in 7 and 8 are fulfilled:

- Field personnel, in jurisdictions where authorized, should start protocols to cease resuscitative efforts or to pronounce death outside the hospital (Class IIa).
- In most US settings, the medical control official must give direct voice-to-voice or on-scene authorization.
- Advance planning for these protocols must occur. The planning should include specific directions for
  —Leaving the body at scene
  —Death certification
  —Transfer to funeral service
  —On-scene family advocate
  —Religious or nondenominational counseling

Reproduced with permission
Guidelines 2000 for Cardiopulmonary Resuscitation and Emergency Cardiovascular Care. *Circulation*, 102(8), 2000. Copyright American Heart Association

Bradycardia Algorithm (Patient is not in cardiac arrest)

Adult Advanced Cardiac Life Support

Bradycardia

- *Slow* (absolute bradycardia = rate <60 bpm)

or

- *Relatively slow* (rate less than expected relative to underlying condition or cause)

Primary ABCD Survey

- Assess ABCs
- Secure airway noninvasively
- Ensure monitor/defibrillator is available

Secondary ABCD Survey

- Assess secondary ABCs (invasive airway management needed?)
- Oxygen–IV access–monitor–fluids
- Vital signs, pulse oximeter, monitor BP
- Obtain and review 12-lead ECG
- Obtain and review portable chest x-ray
- Problem-focused history
- Problem-focused physical examination
- Consider causes (differential diagnoses)

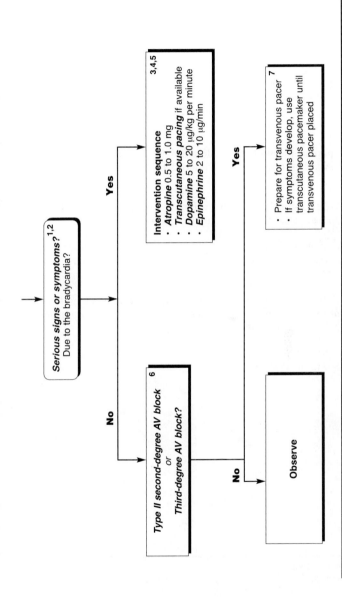

Serious signs or symptoms?[1,2]
Due to the bradycardia?

No / **Yes**

Type II second-degree AV block[6]
or
Third-degree AV block?

Intervention sequence[3,4,5]
- *Atropine* 0.5 to 1.0 mg
- *Transcutaneous pacing* if available
- *Dopamine* 5 to 20 μg/kg per minute
- *Epinephrine* 2 to 10 μg/min

No / **Yes**

Observe

- Prepare for transvenous pacer[7]
- If symptoms develop, use transcutaneous pacemaker until transvenous pacer placed

Notes for Bradycardia Algorithm

1

If the patient has *serious signs* or *symptoms,* make sure they are related to the slow rate.

2

Clinical manifestations include:

- Symptoms (chest pain, shortness of breath, decreased level of consciousness)
- Signs (low blood pressure, shock, pulmonary congestion, congestive heart failure)

3

If the patient is symptomatic, do not delay transcutaneous pacing while awaiting intravenous (IV) access or for *atropine* to take effect.

4

Denervated transplanted hearts will not respond to *atropine.* Go at once to pacing, *catecholamine* infusion, or both.

5

Atropine should be given in repeat doses every 3 to 5 minutes up to a total of 0.03 to 0.04 mg/kg. Use the shorter dosing interval (3 minutes) in severe clinical conditions.

6

Never treat the combination of *third-degree heart block* and *ventricular escape beats* with *lidocaine* (or any agent that suppresses ventricular escape rhythms).

7

Verify patient tolerance and mechanical capture. Use analgesia and sedation as needed.

Pulseless Electrical Activity Algorithm

Adult Advanced Cardiac Life Support

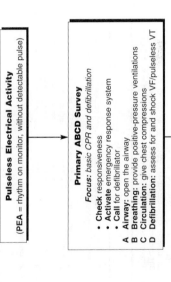

Pulseless Electrical Activity

(PEA = rhythm on monitor, without detectable pulse)

Primary ABCD Survey

Focus: basic CPR and defibrillation

- **Check** responsiveness
- **Activate** emergency response system
- **Call** for defibrillator

A **Airway:** open the airway

B **Breathing:** provide positive-pressure ventilations

C **Circulation:** give chest compressions

D **Defibrillation:** assess for and shock VF/pulseless VT

Secondary ABCD Survey

Focus: more advanced assessments and treatments

A Airway: place airway device as soon as possible
B Breathing: confirm airway device placement by exam plus confirmation device
B Breathing: secure airway device; purpose-made tube holders preferred
B Breathing: confirm effective oxygenation and ventilation
C Circulation: establish IV access
C Circulation: identify rhythm → monitor
C Circulation: administer drugs appropriate for rhythm and condition
C Circulation: assess for occult blood flow ("pseudo-EMT")
D Differential Diagnosis: search for and treat identified reversible causes

---

Review for most frequent causes [1]
(Possible therapies and treatments are given in parentheses)

- Hypovolemia (volume infusion)
- Hypoxia (ventilation)
- Hydrogen ion — acidosis
- Hyper-/hypokalemia
- Hypothermia

- "Tablets" (drug OD, accidents)
- Tamponade, cardiac (pericardiocentesis)
- Tension pneumothorax (needle decompression)
- Thrombosis, coronary (reperfusion therapy)
- Thrombosis, pulmonary embolism (thrombolytics, surgery)

Epinephrine 1 mg IV push, [2] repeat every 3 to 5 minutes

Atropine 1 mg IV (if PEA rate is *slow*), [3] repeat every 3 to 5 minutes as needed, to a total dose of 0.04 mg/kg

Reproduced with permission
Guidelines 2000 for Cardiopulmonary Resuscitation and Emergency Cardiovascular Care. *Circulation*, 102(8), 2000. Copyright American Heart Association

Notes for Pulseless Electrical Activity (PEA) Algorithm

1

Sodium bicarbonate 1 mEq/kg is used as follows:

Class I (acceptable, supported by definitive evidence)

- If patient has known, preexisting hyperkalemia

Class IIa (acceptable, good evidence supports)

- If known, preexisting bicarbonate-responsive acidosis
- In tricyclic antidepressant overdose
- To alkalinize urine in aspirin or other drug overdoses

Class IIb (acceptable, only fair evidence provides support)

- In intubated and ventilated patients with long arrest interval
- On return of circulation, after long arrest interval

May be harmful (Class III) in hypercarbic acidosis

2

Epinephrine: recommended dose is 1 mg intravenous (IV) push every 3 to 5 minutes (Class Indeterminate).

- If this approach fails, higher doses of epinephrine (as much as 0.2 mg/kg) may be used but are not recommended.
- (Although one dose of vasopressin is acceptable for persistent or shock-refractory ventricular fibrillation, we currently lack evidence to support routine use of vasopressin in victims of PEA or asystole.)

3

Atropine: the shorter atropine dose interval (every 3 to 5 minutes) is possibly helpful in cardiac arrest.

- *Atropine* 1 mg IV if electrical activity is *slow* (absolute bradycardia = rate < 60 beats/min) or
- *Relatively slow* (relative bradycardia = rate less than expected, relative to underlying condition)

Index

References in *italics* indicate figures; those followed by t denote tables